A Back and Forth Between Tourism and Health

Tourism and Mobility Systems Set

coordinated by
Philippe Violier

Volume 5

A Back and Forth Between Tourism and Health

From Medical Tourism to Global Health

Sébastien Fleuret

iSTE

WILEY

First published 2022 in Great Britain and the United States by ISTE Ltd and John Wiley & Sons, Inc.

ISTE Ltd
27-37 St George's Road
London SW19 4EU
UK

www.iste.co.uk

John Wiley & Sons, Inc.
111 River Street
Hoboken, NJ 07030
USA

www.wiley.com

Library of Congress Control Number: 2022936845

British Library Cataloguing-in-Publication Data
A CIP record for this book is available from the British Library
ISBN 978-1-78630-538-1

Contents

Introduction

In January 2020, the writing of this book was already well advanced when the first echoes reached us from China of a new virus that seemed to be spreading rapidly and generating serious cases, certainly few in proportion to the number of people affected, but enough to saturate hospital capacities. This was not the first time that such an alert had been issued to the world: SARS in 2002–2003, the H5N1 "bird flu" in 2004 and the A/H1N1 "swine flu" in 2009–2010 were all such alerts where the anticipated catastrophes had failed to materialize. It was therefore with some initial incredulity, but almost a small sense of vindication, that I was considering adding a "Covid-19" section to this book on the interactions between tourism and health. After all, diseases travel in our luggage and this one seemed to be another to add to the list, except that this infection escalated out of all proportion. The world quickly froze, borders were closed, populations were locked down and tourism stopped. The United Nations World Tourism Organization (UNWTO) estimated that in one year of crisis, industry losses amounted to more than 1,000 billion dollars. This was a statistic that was impossible for me to ignore. What should I do? Rewrite the book completely? Adapt it? My decision was to continue the writing and wait until the end before integrating the SARS-CoV-2 disease into the manuscript, depending on the evolution of the pandemic. This took me more than a year, as I had to suspend the writing process in order to prioritize other research and publications related to Covid-19, and, more than a year and a half after the first lockdown in France, the situation remains uncertain. Certainly, vaccines exist, but vaccination campaigns have been slow in countries that do not agree to pay the full price for the doses. Then, after an improvement in the summer of 2021, the arrival of the autumn chill in Europe marked the onset of a fifth epidemic wave. The need for a booster dose of vaccine became apparent. France, which had often procrastinated in its decisions and had not wanted to lock itself down for a third time in January 2021, renewed this decision and is counting on a good rate of vaccination coverage to cope. As for tourism, it started again during the summer of 2020 for a while by adapting, focusing on short journeys and domestic tourism and reconsidering long trips. Then came the crisis and the time of uncertainty before a new recovery the following summer. When will we see the light at the end of the tunnel? History has taught us that global pandemics usually last two to three years at most, less if treatments are available, which is the case with Covid-19. However, this epidemic has provided so many surprises that caution is warranted; nevertheless, this pandemic will end. Therefore, while Covid-19 is a major and impactful event, it should not obscure the complexity of the relationship between tourism and health that pre-existed it and will survive the pandemic, or the fact that health remains largely forgotten in tourism development outside of health crisis episodes. Consequently, the editorial line of this book remains resolutely that which prevailed before the pandemic: the aim is, on the one hand, to present, as broadly as possible, the range of interactions between tourism and health from various perspectives and, on the other hand, to reveal the protean and multiscalar impacts of tourism on health. Covid-19 is specifically covered in Chapter 2 (section 2.1.1).

According to the French Ministry of the Environment, the tourism industry accounts for 9% of global GDP and 6.5% of French GDP (2012), and is directly responsible for the creation of some 900,000 jobs in France. For Stock et al. (2003), the geographical approach to tourism focuses on describing the development of tourist areas, their functioning, their dynamics, the spatial differentiation between tourism factors and the practices of tourism actors and their relationships to space. In other words, tourism reveals both individual and spatialized group practices, influences places, differentiates them from one another and shapes stakeholder interactions. It is therefore a major element of economic development that is highly territorialized, with areas of concentrated activity where direct and indirect effects, environmental impacts and social changes can be observed, all of which fuel the interest in sustainable tourism development. However, there is one component of the sustainability of economic development through tourism that is never addressed: health. It is nowhere to be found, with the notable exception of "medical tourism", or is only mentioned in passing when discussing certain environmental concerns or those related to the well-being of populations. According to a Harris Interaction study (Duhamel 2018), although 90% of French people say they are attentive to the environment and the lives of local populations when they travel, and 70% wish to travel responsibly, sustainable tourism accounts for only 1% of the French market.

However, health can be an interesting lever in a tourism development logic. The number of medical tourists is estimated at around 16 million individuals per year worldwide, representing a turnover exceeding 60 billion dollars and covering geographical areas that capture a significant portion of this market (Latin America, Eastern Europe, India, Southeast Asia) with potentially strong impacts. With regard to the medical profession, first, what happens when trained doctors (and other health professionals) are more interested in the lucrative practice of working for tourists than in working in their local health systems? Then, more broadly, what happens to the health of populations in tourist locations when the healthcare available is more structured towards tourism than towards the local population?

Additionally, it is instructive to examine the way in which promoters of tourism development rely on determinants of health and well-being of populations in order to make health an element in attracting tourism (whether through the environment – air, water, food – or through various so-called "healthy" activities). Territorial marketing is increasingly mobilizing health to increase the attractiveness of certain territories, as part of a broad and global vision of health (Figure I.1).

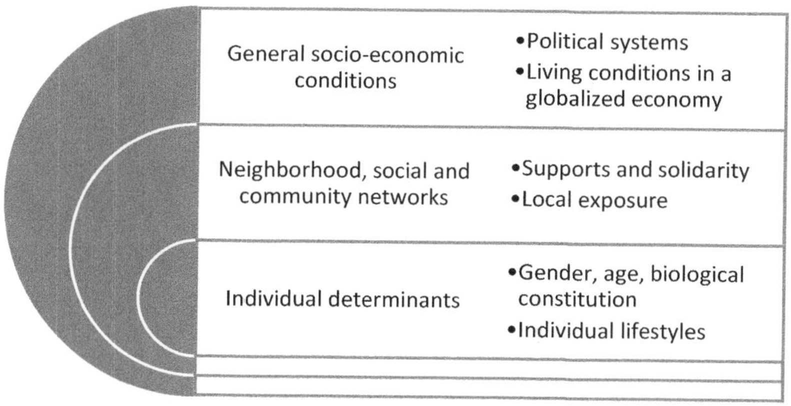

Figure I.1. *Determinants of health, simplified diagram from Dahlgren and Whitehead (1991)*

"Individual determinants" of health refers to personal factors which, when aggregated, produce what is known in epidemiology as compositional effects. Thus, a tourist population composed mainly of senior citizens does not pose the same challenges as a population of young spring breakers, for example. "Individual lifestyles" refers to the behavior of tourists, on the one hand (do they comply with prevention messages? Do they take precautions or expose themselves by taking risks?), and to the changes in lifestyles that result from confrontations between receptive local societies and visitors with different habits, on the other (all the more so where the initial differences between lifestyles and living standards is great).

At the neighborhood (local) level, social and community networks strongly determine health. Travel is a temporary separation from these supports, which can pose health problems. Within host societies, tourism can lead to a transformation of social relationships and, sometimes, to the ex nihilo (re)construction of a place. It then takes time to build support networks, which are essential for health, in new territories that are shaped by tourism (see, for example, Cabezas 2008).

Finally, “general socio-economic conditions” refers to systems organization: the globalized system of the travel and tourism industry, national health systems and more localized systems of territorial planning form a general framework in which the interactions between tourism and health are many but unstated.

Structured into five chapters, this book proposes to pass back and forth between tourism and health in order to catalog the interactions that exist between these two sectors and to discuss the issues at stake. In this way, the importance of taking health into account in tourism development will be highlighted.

1

Tourism and Health, a Long-standing and Renewed Relationship

First quoted in the 19th century, the word tourism referred to "a journey relating to a Grand Tour and the mobility of 'health' towards spa towns" (Duhamel 2018). This was well before the advent of the so-called leisure society and the development of mass tourism. The Grand Tour then was a male practice of educational travel across Europe, reserved for the aristocracy, which led the young notables who engaged in it to put the finishing touches on their education, and to tour certain high places, the premises of the great tourist destinations.

The main destinations of the Grand Tour were France (from Calais to Paris – a must – then to the Alps and/or Provence), Germany (Munich, Frankfurt, Berlin and even the shores of the Baltic Sea), Switzerland (Geneva) and especially Italy (Venice, Milan, Pisa, Florence, Rome, Naples, and so on). Some ventured to the Iberian Peninsula or to Greece and the Middle East, but this required up to five years of travel and a substantial family fortune.

Some famous writers such as Johann Wolfgang von Goethe and Alexandre Dumas took the Grand Tour, with its benefits described as being, above all, cultural and personal. The first of these benefits was to make friends and build up an international social network that could potentially be useful for a military or diplomatic career, for example. Works of art (such as statues and paintings) were also purchased, thus contributing to the circulation of culture and artistic trends. The Grand Tour promoted the diffusion of neoclassicism in Europe. On a more personal level, it was an opportunity to strengthen skills, to build self-confidence, to learn what

For a color version of all the figures in this chapter, see: www.iste.co.uk/fleuret/tourism.zip.

constituted "good manners" in different countries, as well as to develop sexual education, albeit at the risk of certain diseases.

Around the same time, winter tourism developed, which consisted of seeking a milder and more temperate climate, as well as, if possible, good sea air in order to escape the harsh winters of northern Europe. This is how, for example, a wintering community of British people in Nice raised funds to build a resort path that has now become the famous Promenade des Anglais (a promenade associated with sea bathing or spa treatment was considered to be beneficial for health).

To understand these phenomena, we must place ourselves in the context of the time. The medical and hygienic discourse that developed in the 19th century was accompanied by a rejection of the town and its miasmas. Doctors lauded the benefits of nature, pure air, sea or alpine air, water, etc. A plethora of guides and works codified therapy through resorts or treatment.

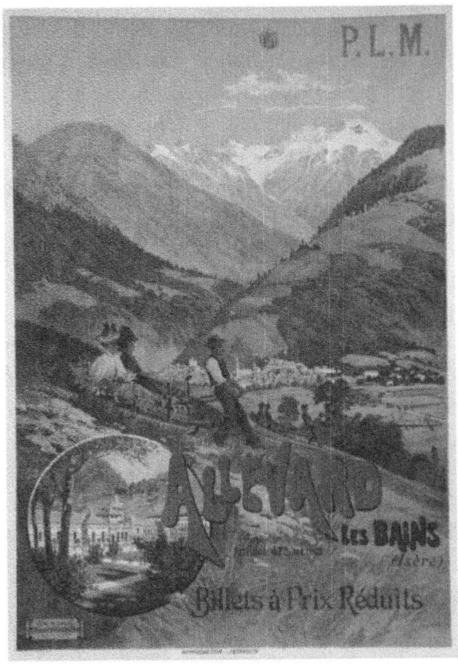

Figure 1.1. *Advertisement for the Paris–Lyon–Marseille railroads (19th century) (source: INA)*

It was only following a long process (Chessex 1997; Bertrand 2010), stimulated by the development of the railroad (Figure 1.1), that the practice of tourism was democratized on initial foundations largely linked to preoccupations with health. Then, little by little, bathers discovered the joys of the beach, and travelers in search of relaxation sought worldly distractions in the palaces and casinos that flourished to meet this new demand.

Thus, the medical discourse strongly contributed to the development of travel and vacationing practices and, by extension, to the birth of tourist resorts. However, while it effectively developed during the 19th century, the origins of this phenomenon date back to ancient history.

1.1. From Hippocrates to thermalism

As a primitive form of tourist travel, mobility towards the spa towns certainly, historically, wove the first links between tourism and health. In ancient times, medicine and religion were intertwined. It was Hippocrates who laid the first foundations of modern medicine, notably through his treatise *On Airs, Waters and Places*, in which he advocated the systematic observation of climatic and hydrological conditions and lifestyle habits, particularly dietary habits, in the places where the disciples of the School of Kos were to practice their medicine. Through these propositions, he introduced the notion of the systematic observation of the conditions of appearance of a pathology and, in so doing, distinguished between the environmental or behavioral origins of diseases and a divine origin linked to beliefs. Following Hippocrates' recommendations, it was no longer a question of moving from one place to another according to the seasons to escape from bad conditions (a form of nomadism), or of going on a pilgrimage to a spa, but, for example, to get away from the city in search of fresh mountain air and sunshine. The locations of the Greek sanctuaries and places of convalescence testify to a consideration of the environment and the climate. The presence of the sea was already a notable factor in Kos, the Mecca of the Hippocratic school.

1.1.1. *The Roman period*

The Romans also developed second homes, which were often coastal. Rome was known to be unhealthy in summer and was deserted by the wealthy classes who retired to the nearby Apennines which, despite their low elevation, offered milder temperatures. The quality of the air and water in these secondary villas was reputed to be better, as evidenced by the habits of Cicero, for instance, who would retire to his villa in Tusculum (20 km from Rome and 670 m above sea level) when he suffered from an upset stomach.

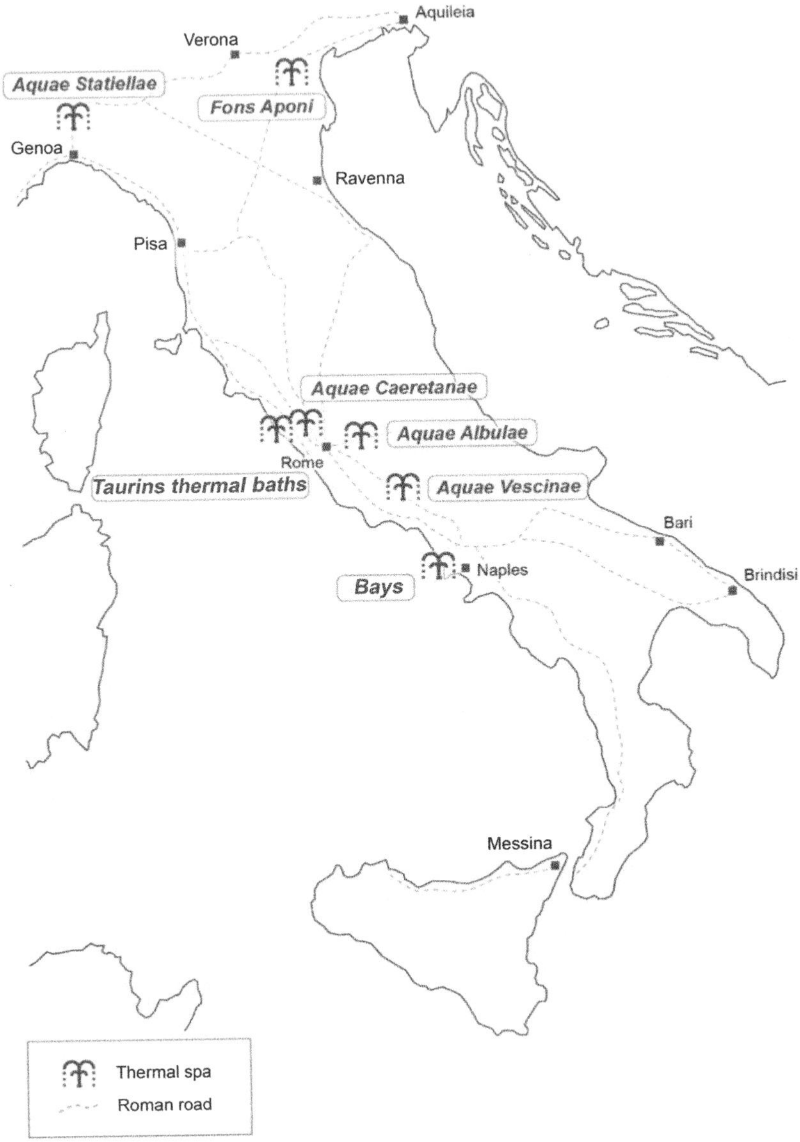

Figure 1.2. *The main thermal centers of the Roman period (source: according to Guérin-Beauvois (2000))*

At that time, the pharmacopoeia available to doctors was limited and thermal waters and muds had already been identified for their therapeutic virtues, but in connection with divinities who were often identified as protectors of thermal springs. Priests were the first hydrologists! The remains of ex-voto offerings and fragments found near the thermal baths have provided archaeologists with indications of the pathologies treated (some of these remains are sculptures representing treated organs). We find testimonies on the interest of taking thermal baths in the writings of Aristotle, Plutarch and Galen.

The Roman Empire placed great emphasis on thermal baths, and Pliny the Elder and Herodotus described the first principles of crenotherapy through a reflection on the duration of treatments, the best season to carry them out, the different types of baths, and so on.

In addition to the daily practice of bathing in the city or in the richest villas, there were treatments that combined the therapeutic principle of water use with recreational practices and festive or sports activities. "It was therefore a question of the acts that constituted treatment: hygiene and body care, but also appeasement of the spirit, relaxation and sociability, all activities within the framework in which thermal man evolved, as much in antiquity as nowadays" (Guérin-Beauvois 2000).

In Gaul, therapeutic uses of the springs were already widespread but were to develop during the Gallo-Roman period. These springs were protected by the thermal deity Borvo, whose name is composed of two evocative Celtic words: *berw* (which means hot, boiling) and *von* (which means fountain). We can detect these terms in the etymology of certain thermal spas, such as La Bourboule. Other places would develop later under Roman influence and inherit Latin toponyms linked to water, Aix-les-Bains, for example (Aquae Gratianae).

1.1.2. *Elsewhere in the world*

While the Greeks and Romans were pioneers in Western history, the search for beneficial waters was not the prerogative of the Europeans. Historical forms of thermal tourism have been found in Asia, for example.

In the center of China, one example is the Huaqing Hot Springs at the foot of Mount Li, near the modern-day city of Xi'an, whose first thermal pools date back to the Qin dynasty (221–206 BCE). This was a resort for the emperors and their court during the subsequent Han dynasty (206 BCE to 220 CE) and later the Tang dynasty (618 to 907 CE), who built a palace around an artificial pool. The site was then taken over by Taoist monks who built several temples. In 1936, Chiang Kai-shek was captured there by the communists and released on the condition that he promised to collaborate against their common enemy, the Japanese invader. Finally, the communist regime developed a spa there (still in operation) in order to offer treatments to the workers of the nation. Thanks to this thermal and historical past, this site has now become a tourist and heritage site.

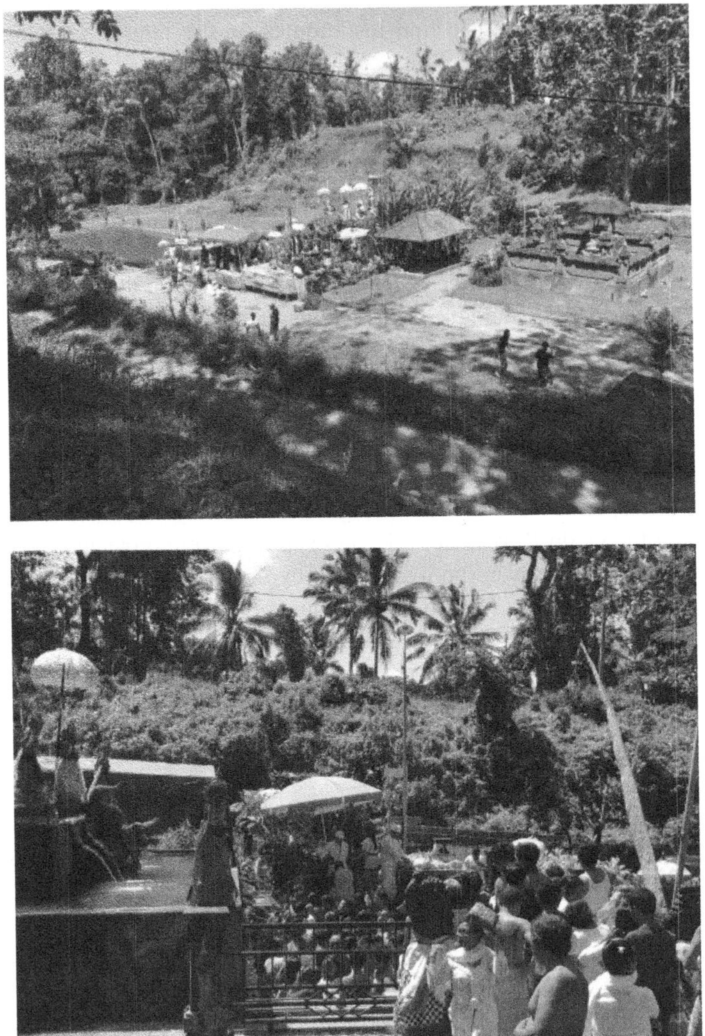

Figure 1.3. *Ceremony at the Tamba Waras Temple baths (photos: S. Fleuret 2016)*

In Bali, Indonesia, the tradition of purification through bathing gave rise to the construction of numerous sacred temples around springs and pools, which, in addition to their attractiveness for the spiritual tourism of the locals, constitute a heritage attraction for international tourists. In some places, bathing is authorized for international tourists, whereas in others (Figure 1.3), internal Indonesian tourism has developed in connection with ceremonies.

In Latin America, also, thermalism is the basis for the attractiveness of certain sites, in connection with volcanism. This is the case, for example, in Cajamarca, a which includes Los Banõs del Inca (the Baths of the Inca) District. This modern-day coastal resort in the north of the Andes is probably the most famous in Peru: its waters are rich in chloride and sulfur and gush out at a temperature of 70°C. Since the Inca period, the therapeutic properties attributed to these waters have been used in the treatment of bone and nervous system disorders. The stone bathtub in which, according to legend, the Inca Atahualpa bathed before confronting Pizzaro, is preserved as a testament to a past that some archaeologists have traced back a millennium.

1.1.3. *To the Middle Ages, then in the Renaissance*

The medieval period in the West saw the Hippocratic concepts stifled by religious dogma, and pilgrimages for health reasons faded for a number of centuries. However, at the same time, in the Arab world, physicians such as Avicenna and Averroes advocated mobility towards certain regions for people suffering from pulmonary and tubercular diseases: Avicenna proposed Crete, while Averroes recommended the hot and dry air of Egypt or Ethiopia.

In the 16th century, a schism between the Church of Rome and England caused the decline of pilgrimages whose purpose was spiritual fulfillment and which were condemned by Protestantism. Pilgrimage became introspective, without the need for mobility, but the quest for fulfilment remained and gradually shifted to the search for bodily fulfilment through healthy lifestyles and particularly through travel to spa destinations, with the goal being physical healing (Duhamel 2018). The coastal resorts became "healthy places", and doctors prescribed bathing in the sea as a remedy for all sorts of ailments.

The Hippocratic trend re-emerged with the Renaissance, accompanied, in the cities, by the development of hygienism and the invention of epidemiology. In Europe, there was a renewed interest in water, which, with the advent of sanitized urbanism, was no longer simply a vector of diseases.

The example of Bath, a spa town since Roman times, is a model of its type. Before becoming a popular tourist center in the 17th and 18th centuries, Bath still largely resembled a medieval city, surrounded by ramparts and narrow streets.

John Woods was the architect responsible for the city's transformation, and although much of his design was never realized, his work laid the foundation for Bath's transformation into the Georgian city that became the recreational capital of England and a model for other spas. Yet, the city did not originally have much going for it beyond its baths, only an abbey and a declining trade. It is its status as a spa town that has shaped its development and its recognition as a major destination. The integration of historical remains, notably its Roman baths into its Georgian architecture, has contributed to this success, which is now reflected in the site's Unesco World Heritage listing.

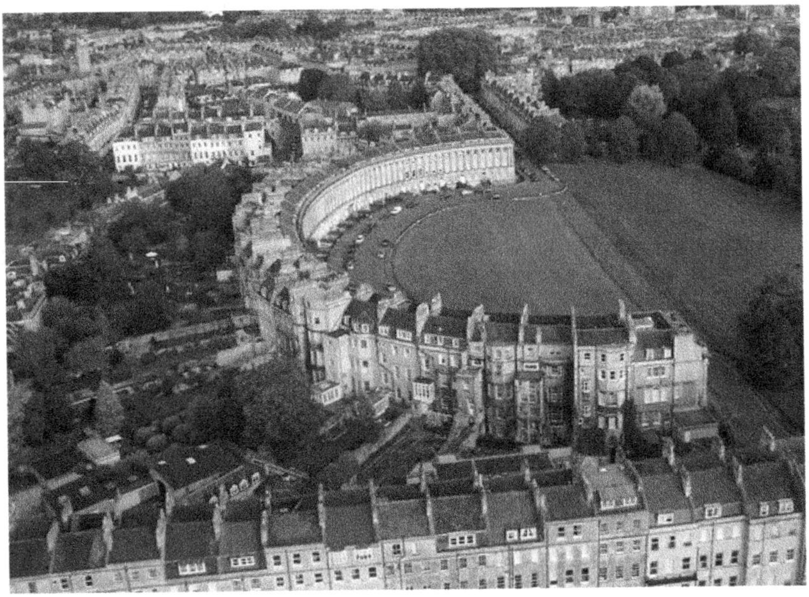

Figure 1.4. *The Royal Crescent Hotel in Bath (source: geograph.org.uk)*

Among Bath's architectural symbols is The Circus, inspired by the Colosseum in Rome in an attempt to recreate a small palatine in the center of Bath with the adjacent Queen Square and a forum that was never built. The three orders (Doric, Roman and Corinthian) are superimposed on the curved façade of this building. The Royal Crescent Hotel (Figure 1.4), designed by Woods' son, follows the same inspiration. Other emblematic buildings related to health mark the architectural landscape of

Bath, such as the Royal National Hospital for Rheumatic Diseases. Thus, welcoming the aristocracy for treatment shaped the architecture of these buildings, and it was the same in other cities around Europe.

The Belgian resort of Spa, launched by the English at the end of the 18th century and based on the Bath model, was also successful in that its name has become the generic term describing thermal resorts and bathing facilities. Following these successes, the principal monarchies around the continent followed England's lead and founded their own spas: Baden-Baden near Stuttgart, Karlovy Vary (Karlsbad) and Mariánské Lázně (Marienbad) in Bohemia, Montecatini in Tuscany, Aix-les-Bains in Savoy, and Bagnères-de-Luchon and Vichy in France (Lecler 2008).

1.1.4. *Modern history of spa towns*

Bad Rothenfelde in Germany is another example, somewhat different from Bath, but equally interesting. In 1724, an underground salt water spring was discovered there. In order to exploit the salt, a wall (*Gradierwerk*) about 500 m long and 20 m high, a wooden frame with thin blackthorn branches and twigs, was built (Figure 1.5). There are approximately 50 *Gradierwerke* in Germany and a few in Austria and Poland. This very open structure made it possible to heat the water in a basin at the top (Figure 1.6) and then, by making the water flow towards its base (Figure 1.7), provoke partial evaporation (the structure being well ventilated) and increase the concentration of salt from 6 to 20%, facilitating its subsequent collection. However, it turned out that this wall had a secondary effect, that of purifying the surrounding air. An activity was therefore developed related to the inhalation of this air purified by the salt water. After the closure of the salt works in 1969, the site became known as an Inhalatorium and attracted visitors from Lower Saxony and Rhineland-Westphalia, as much for this as for the city's treatment activity, which had been developed since 1908 with the creation of salt baths and a spa.

In Bad Rothenfelde, good water and good air are the basis of hygiene and are generally associated with urban planning, but – unjustly – not so much with tourism.

To complete this commentary on the uses of water in an approach combining health and tourism, let us expand upon our last case: the town of Évian-les-Bains, on the edge of Lake Geneva, a thermal and tourist resort where an industry has been developed around the commercialization of mineral water.

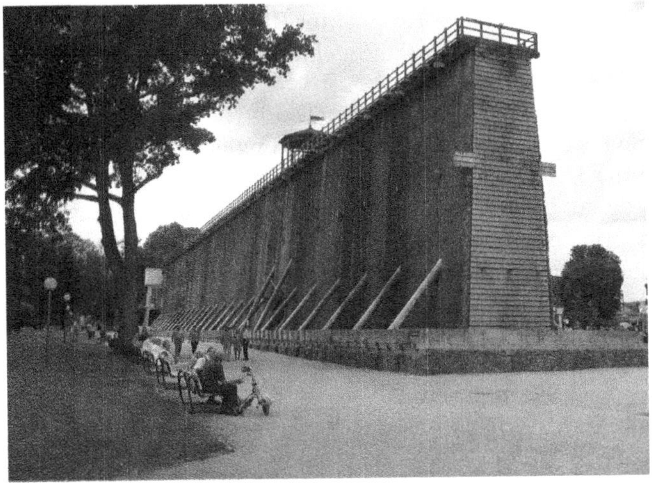

Figure 1.5. *The Gradierwerke at Bad Rothenfelde (source: zoover.com)*

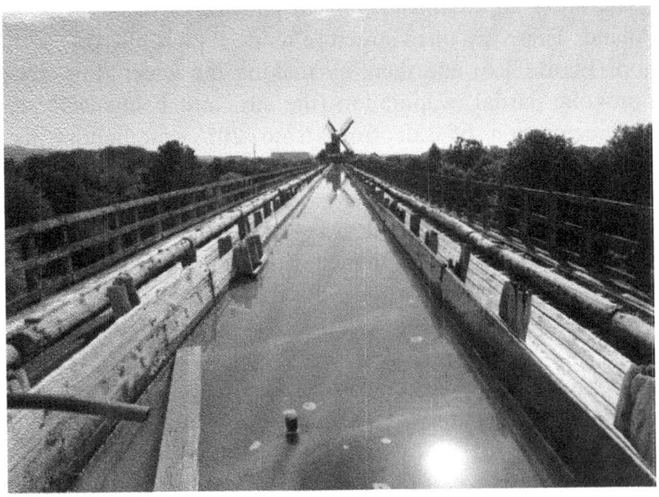

Figure 1.6. *Evaporation basin on top of the structure (source: Osnabrueckerland.de)*

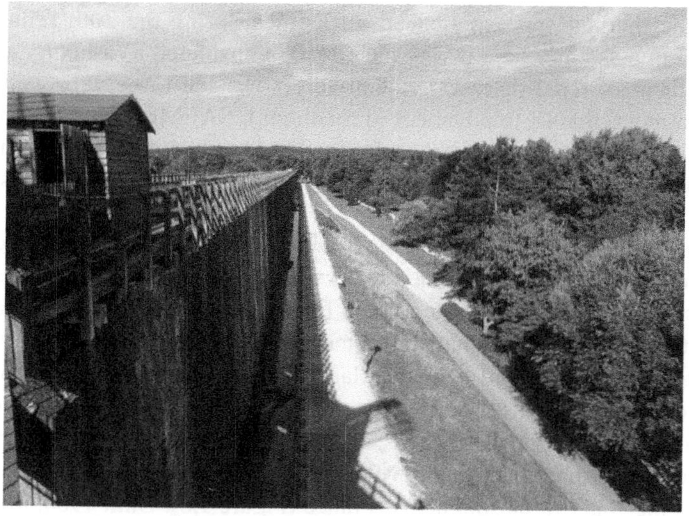

Figure 1.7. *Runoff along the walls (source: Osnabrueckerland.de)*

Évian was, first of all, one of the favorite places of the nobility of Chablais (province of Thonon-les-Bains), who were attracted by the waters of the ferruginous spring of a neighboring city, Amphion. The sovereigns of Sardinia and their court made frequent visits there before the attachment of Savoy to France, which gave the region an international reputation. At the same time, at the end of the 18th century, the curative virtues of the water from the Cachat spring in Évian itself were discovered. Medical recognition was just around the corner, as Jules Cottet, a doctor at the resort, established the principles of a cure for diuresis and proved the relationship between a large intake of pure water and improvement in kidney function. A shift took place, and the bathers became patients. Since Amphion had no accommodation capacity, Évian replaced it and developed as a tourist and spa resort. In 1826, a bathing facility was built there, and some modest equipment including about 30 residences. The annexation of Savoy by France in 1860 brought about a period of development that resulted in the construction of rich residences on the shores of Lake Geneva and the acquisition of a status as a center of global importance, highly prized by the Parisian upper middle class. Tourism had an impact on urban planning: the lakefront was developed with a promenade – bathing and walking formed the basis of the treatment – and in 1865, a casino was built to entertain this clientele. The same year, an imperial decree consecrated the vocation of the resort by granting it the name of Évian-les-Bains and, in 1881, a railway station was built following an agreement between the Paris–Lyon–Marseille (PLM) railway company and the *Société Anonyme des Eaux Minérales d'Évian* (SAEME). From then on, the railroad served the resort, encouraging an influx of visitors.

While the thermal spa experienced difficulties during the 20th century (it had been locked in a sector where it was specifically considered as a luxury and limited to the treatment of renal diseases, which were now able to be very well cared for without treatment, thanks to advances in medicine), SAEME, initially conceived on the back of tourism development, was destined to literally "define the French bottled mineral water market" (Watin-Augouard 2002) and to write its own success story[1].

The story is as follows. Escaping the French Revolution, the Marquis of Lessert, suffering from kidney stones, decided to go to Amphion to take the waters and treat his kidneys. By pure chance, he stopped in Évian and quenched his thirst at a spring belonging to a certain Mr. Cachat and found the water he drank there pleasant, light and easy to drink. He came back regularly and found himself cured, which was proven following a medical report. Mr. Cachat saw this as a great opportunity, fenced in his spring and began to market his water under the name Evian-Cachat. At the beginning of the 20th century, the development of the glass bottle and the aluminum cap allowed the water to be sold across France (Figure 1.8). Until 1960, it was sold in pharmacies as alkaline mineral water, recommended for diets. The growth of supermarkets provided an outlet for the brand which, in the 1970s, came under the control of the BSN brand (now the Danone group). The strength of the Evian mineral water brand lies in its ability to use both contextual factors and strong, ideally targeted communication messages. The context was the development of tourism, a quest for natural spaces and waters in the 18th century, and then the extension of these aspirations in the face of growing urbanization (cities need to be supplied with water) and its attendant pollution and other frenetic lifestyles. Communication was initially focused on health benefits, the message at the end of the 19th century being that Evian-Source-Cachat was "the most effective diet water and the best table water" (slogan of the time). In the 1930s, the argument of bacterial purity took over: mineral water is sterile, which makes it an excellent bottled water that does not need to be boiled. Then, a change of direction took place when the spa industry entered into crisis, and the number of curists stagnated and even declined. Evian refocused on its origins, and the brand reused the arguments and visual references that had made the place attractive to tourists; except that instead of bringing the tourist to the destination, it was the destination that came to the tourist, in a bottle and with promises in the form of slogans: "*L'eau d'Evian, issue des Alpes, a le goût délicieux des sources de montagne*" (Evian water, from the Alps, has the delicious taste of mountain springs), "*Boire Evian, c'est respirer à 3 000 mètres*" (Drinking Evian is like breathing at 3,000 m), "*L'eau d'Evian vous donne ce que les Alpes lui ont donné*" (Evian water gives you what the Alps have given it), "*L'eau que vous buvez est aussi importante que l'air que vous respirez*" (The water you drink is as important as the air you breathe), etc.

1 http://www.prodimarques.com/sagas_marques/evian/evian.php (accessed March 29, 2021).

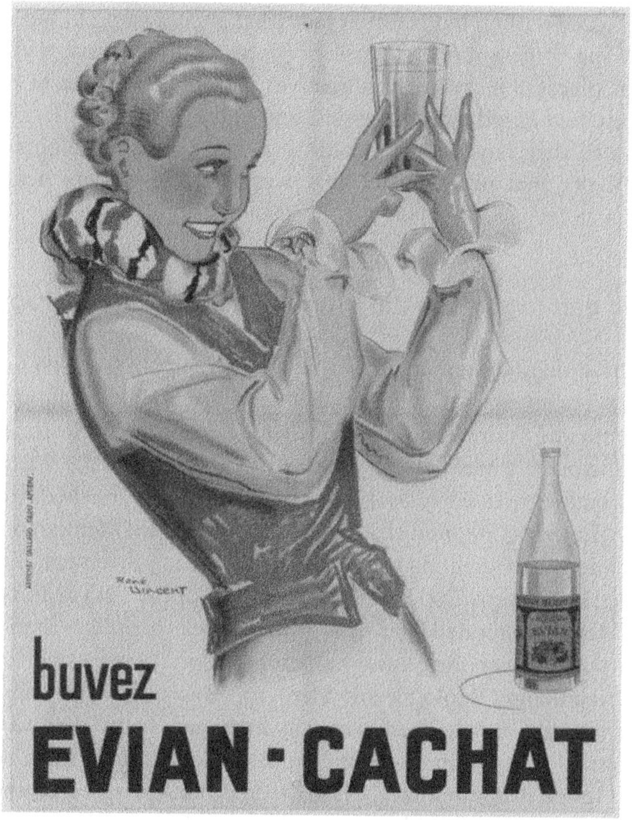

Figure 1.8. *Advertisement for Evian water, 1930 (source: gallica.bnf.fr)*

With this image of a natural product with healthy properties conferred on it by mountains, Evian water accompanied the evolution of a consumer society that increasingly questioned the quality and healthy or harmful nature of what it was ingesting. In the mid-1980s, it promoted the product's physiological properties with the slogan "*La force de l'équilibre*" (The power of equilibrium) and the promise of visible effects on the body: "*Je bois Evian et ça se voit*" (I drink Evian and it shows). From there, under the direction of advertisers, Evian began to systematically use babies, animated by computer graphics, to convey the idea, through television commercials, that "Drinking pure water balanced in minerals every day maintains your body's youth", and like a return to the origins of thermalism, we return to the idea of a fountain of youth.

Beyond the success of an industrial brand, what is interesting in the story of Evian is the interweaving of geography (its use of places and their imagery), tourism (the frequentation of places that makes it attractive) and the development of an industry that markets a product based on these assets, and in the example of Evian, we find all the uses of water that have made health a factor in the development of tourist destinations: "Water that heals, water that washes and protects health" (Bruston 2000).

1.2. From sea bathing to coastal tourism and thalassotherapy

There is thus a long heritage that has shaped the reputation of spa towns to which curative virtues are attributed without the need for medicalization, such as the fountains of youth and "miraculous" springs which constitute milestones or stages of pilgrimages. However, a new factor emerged at the end of the 18th century: the practice of sea bathing. As early as 1769, Hugues Maret published *Mémoire sur la manière d'agir des bains de mer et leurs usages vivifiants* (Memoir on the way sea bathing works and its invigorating uses), discussing the improvement of rheumatism in particular (quoted by Vincent (2007)). At the beginning of the 19th century, Dieppe and Boulogne-sur-Mer inaugurated the first French sea bathing establishments for therapeutic purposes. Over the years, numerous resorts were established along the French coast, including Boulogne-sur-Mer, La Rochelle, Cherbourg, Deauville, Arcachon, Biarritz and Cannes. There were "hydrotherapy baths" or "wave baths" that were always carried out within a medical framework: immersions in seawater were timed and only lasted a few minutes. "Bathers and doctors agree on the three major qualities required of the sea: coldness or at least freshness, salinity and turbulence. Pleasure is born from water that lashes us. The bather delights when he experiences the weight of the ocean's immense forces" (Corbin 2018).

A large number of scientific works by doctors were published to codify the practice of bathing and to highlight the care and therapeutic benefits that it could bring, depending on the diseases. "These guides constitute true geographical classifications of seawater and consequently highlight coastal resorts, with each doctor extolling the benefits of their own seawater compared with others" (Bertaud 2012; see Box 1.1).

> Dr. Pouget, physician-inspector of the Royan sea baths, naturally advocated the Royan coast in his book *Recherches et observations sur l'emploi hygiénique et médical de l'eau de mer et sur les influences de l'atmosphère maritime* (Research and observations on the hygiene and medical use of sea water and on the influences of sea air), published in 1851. Dr. L. Gigot-Suard wrote that he would not have produced his guide, published in 1860, if he "only had to repeat to the reader what has been said in all the bathing manuals. However, through the happy and exceptional disposition of its beaches, Royan offers

resources to therapeutics and hygiene that cannot be found elsewhere." Gigot-Suard favored the gentle undulations of Grande-Conche rather than the agitation of the sea at Pontaillac: "While at Grand-Conche the movements of the water are extremely moderate, so that bathers receive only a very weak wave, at Pontaillac on the contrary, it is a real wave with its jolts, percussions and shocks. Between these two extremes, we still find intermediate degrees on the conches of Foncillon and Chaiz." At the same time, in 1862, Dr. Salmon, a colleague but competitor of Gigot-Suard, wrote his booklet, *Coup d'œil médico-philosophique sur l'emploi de l'eau de mer* (Brief medico-philosophical look at the use of sea water). This doctor, who was attached to the hydrotherapy establishment of the Royan casino, wrote that "sea water is administered in an infinite variety of ways, each of which requires sustained care and particular attention, the omission or negligence of which can compromise the success of this energetic and often heroic medication. Thus, outside: (1) the cold bath, taken at sea, under the exciting and tonic action of waves; (2) the bathtub bath, pure or mixed, at temperatures which should vary depending on the cases, that is, according to lesions which are to be combatted; (3) the cold affusion, exerted on the totality of the body; (4) top-down showers; (5) foot baths; (6) lotions; (7) various local applications; (8) sweating, with its various modes and degrees; (9) pulverization, with its multiple conditions. [...] Among the resorts we visited, there are many that lack hydrotherapy equipment and very few of them offer more complete and better established equipment than in Royan. In Dieppe, as in Trouville, Le Havre and Fécamp, there is only a single beach, while in Royan there are three, maybe four, in which the agitation of sea waves presents different degrees, hence different modes of action, a circumstance of great interest for the treatment of illnesses, according to the measure of tonicity that one wishes to produce or provoke."

Box 1.1. *The therapeutics of sea baths (translated extract from Bertaud (2012))*

Bathing was not permitted without supervision, especially for women: the bather's guide set the bathing times and administered immersion, plunging the head of the bather at the top of the waves and keeping it under water in order to generate a suffocation, which was considered therapeutic. Men were able to benefit from more autonomy, and their bathing guide's main function was to advise and guarantee their safety.

The first sea baths were thus battles against the elements, "a fight against engulfment" (Corbin 2018). The dimension of pleasure, of basking or of communion with the elements through swimming intervened later in history, and moreover, in a trend concomitant with the development of sports practices, was aimed at maintaining a healthy body and mind. Thus, coastal tourism progressively evolved from its initial form of asceticism through cold baths to become a recreational pleasure time, as described by P. Morand in his book *Bains de mers* (Sea bathing) in

1960. The three S model – sea, sand and sun – was born and led to bodily hedonism (Duhamel 2018), on which we will return later in this book.

The advent of pleasure bathing and relaxing seaside tourism relegated therapeutic activities to the confines of thalassotherapy establishments. Thus, we come full circle: the quest for water, whether sea water (thalassotherapy) or spring water (balneotherapy) in the context of therapeutic practices, is nowadays included within the term crenotherapy. At this stage of our analysis, it is advisable to take the time to differentiate between medical thermalism and thalassotherapy, which, although having common origins, today constitute two distinct families.

1.2.1. *Thermal medicine*

The practices of thermal medicine are recognized as complementary medicines in France, where 12 therapeutic orientations for thermal cures have been defined by the social security[2] and may possibly lead to treatment if prescribed by a doctor. At the European level, the recognition of these treatments is also progressing (Canista 2015). The treatments provided are of two types: external (such as showers, water baths, mud baths, massages, etc.) and internal hydrotherapy (drink cures, inhalations, and so on). The website of the French National Council of Thermal Establishments (*Conseil National des Etablissements Thermaux*, CNETh) highlights a number of supporting scientific studies.

These cures can be prescribed as well as, or as a complement to, certain treatments, in particular chemotherapy or heavy anti-inflammatory treatments in the care of rheumatism, for example. Today in France, there are 600,000 people taking spa treatments and 10 million days of treatment per year (2018) across the 110 French spa establishments (spread over 90 spas; see Figure 1.9). A spa treatment consists of thermal mud applications and freshwater treatments: thermal water jets, high-pressure showers, submerging, steam rooms, massages and hydromassages, walking sessions in a swimming pool, and so on. It may be accompanied by tourist activities in the surrounding areas, as treatments generally last only two to three hours per day.

2 Source: https://www.medecinethermale.fr/curistes/en-pratique/orientations-therapeutiques.html (accessed on August 16, 2019).

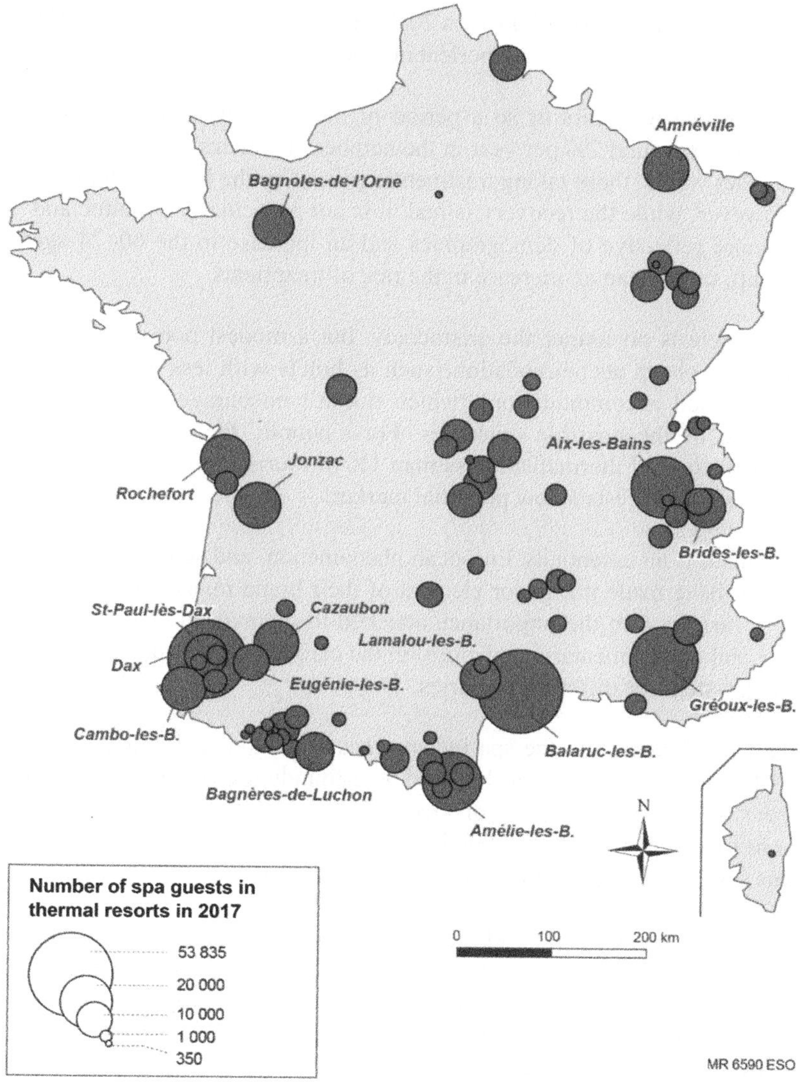

Figure 1.9. *Thermal treatment establishments in France and their capacities (source: www.location-cure.net 2017; Conseil National des Etablissements Thermaux 2021; design and production: Fleuret S., Lepetit A., UMR 6590 ESO)*

Two-thirds of clients are over 60 years old, and the efforts of spa towns to rejuvenate their clientele and their image through offers oriented more towards fitness and sport than towards treatment have not been met with the expected success.

According to CNETh (2015), following a 20% drop in attendance during the 1990s and 2000s, the spa industry has been experiencing the following:

> for the last ten years or so a period of measured dynamism, with a growth of around 2% per year in the number of patients under contract; in other words, those taking treatments covered by the health insurance. However, while the recovery is real, it is not particularly dynamic and is more reflective of demographics and an increase in the 60–74 age group, rather than an increase in the rate of treatments.

The clientele is no longer the aristocracy, but a modest population which will often prioritize cheap accommodation (such as hotels with less than three stars, or private, furnished accommodation), which doesn't encourage them to extend an offer in spite of the possible outcomes. For example, the current poor level of internationalization of thermalism (less than 1% of tourists in French establishments are international) suggests a new potential market.

Thermalism is an essentially European phenomenon, and some major cities, such as Budapest, have made it a major element of their brand image. We have observed significant variations in the importance attached to thermalism (and more widely to alternative and complementary medicines) in the care (curative) and social protection (insurance) systems of different countries.

In the United Kingdom, the spa industry has undergone a major crisis, although the city of Bath has continued to be cited as a founding example of water tourism. During the International Festival of Geography at Saint-Dié-des-Vosges in 2000, Marc Lohez (2000b) made the following observation: "The most prestigious of the spa towns saw [...] its eponymous activity disappearing in the 1970s [author's note: this was in 1978], a victim of the mistrust of British doctors. The National Health Service withdrew its approval and the UK spa industry, deprived of social security benefits, went out of business." With its architectural heritage and history dating back to Roman times, the city maintained its tourist appeal, but it was not until 2006 that the royal baths were reopened, testifying to a renewed interest in gentler approaches to medicine and care.

Conversely, in Eastern Europe, thermalism is particularly valued and was the object of significant research investment in the former USSR. Today, Russia still has a Scientific Center for Restorative Medicine and Balneotherapy (Persianova-Dubrova et al. 2012) and a scientific journal, the *Journal of Physiotherapy, Balneology and Rehabilitation*.

Elsewhere in the world, thermalism is less prevalent; there are only approximately 20 spa centers in the United States, for example.

1.2.2. *Thalassotherapy*

Thalassotherapy centers are, by their very nature, located by the sea and use natural sea water for its various virtues: rich in minerals and trace elements (such as magnesium, potassium, sodium, calcium, silicon and fluorine), it also contains microorganisms with, for instance, antibacterial, antiviral and hormonal properties.

Various types of treatments are offered by thalassotherapy centers: hydrotherapy using heated sea water (such as hydromassage baths), algotherapy using seaweed poultices enriched with essential oils and dry treatments in the form of various massage treatments. Thalassotherapy centers are a mix between a tourist accommodation, with its hotel functions, and a healthcare establishment. In the field there are doctors, physiotherapists, hydrotherapists, dieticians and beauticians. In the thermal spas previously mentioned, in addition to curative treatments, are purely tourist activities relating to water (spa relaxation), wellness (sports activities), the mind (workshops and conferences) or simply the discovery of the region and its beauty, like any other tourist destination.

In contrast to spa resorts, which have experienced an economic slump and an aging clientele, thalassotherapy centers appear to be in good health according to the In Extenso TCH – France Thalasso Thalassotherapy Observatory (2017), with an increase in revenues and relatively stable attendance. The clientele is primarily domestic, and there seems to be a clear distinction between tourists looking for simple relaxation, who will visit hotels with non-medical spas, and tourists looking for a specific treatment who will not hesitate to pay more for treatment in a specialized establishment. The list of ailments treated at the 50 or so centers in France (Figure 1.10) is long. Personalized treatment programs found on the Internet include those for: back and joint pain, getting back into shape after childbirth, menopause support, programs for resuming sports activity, relaxation and even help with quitting smoking!

The distinction between a thalassotherapy center and a thermal spa is that, while the former is limited to one establishment, the latter is an entire city. Thalassotherapy centers are, however, systematically positioned within tourist destinations that offer other seaside attractions (such as beaches and marine leisure activities).

Over time, since the emergence of the phenomenon in France during the second half of the 20th century, we have seen an evolution in thalassotherapy centers, from an initially highly medicalized approach (functional rehabilitation centers) to less medicalized centers, with a sports focus (thalassotherapy institutes) and finally, more recently, more luxurious and even less medicalized "thalasso-spas". This shift seems to be going hand in hand with the evolution of the touristification of the destinations that host thalassotherapy centers. When the health argument, on which the phenomenon is based, is no longer sufficient to ensure its sustainability, it is the broader argument of well-being that is put forward.

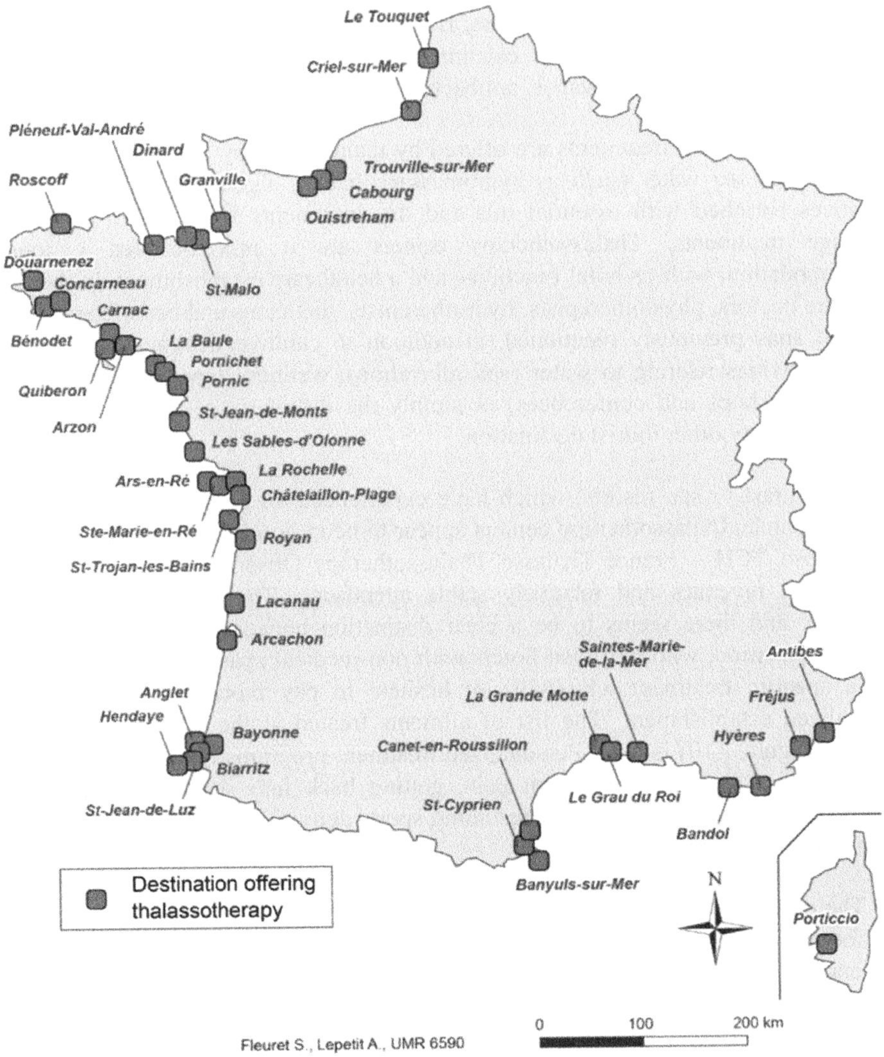

Figure 1.10. *Thalassotherapy centers (source: France Thalasso; Thalasso-line; Thalazur 2021; design and production: Fleuret S., Lepetit A., UMR 6590)*

1.3. Fresh air, nature, health and tourism

Climate and health had long-established links with travel, long before the invention of the word tourism, and there is evidence dating back to the 3rd millennium BCE of mobilities for curative reasons (Kevan 1993), probably in the form of pilgrimages.

Evidence of consideration of the impact of atmospheric factors[3] on health can be found in the practices of Mesopotamian, Egyptian, Chinese and Indian physicians in antiquity. In an article entitled "Quests for cures: A history of tourism for climate and health", Kevan (1993) attributes the first known statement by a physician of the need to undertake seasonal migrations for health reasons to the Indian sage Sustra (600 to 500 BCE):

> He [Sustra] pointed out that Varsah (the rainy period from mid-July to mid-September) was an unhealthy time of year and suggested that rulers should move their courts away from the cities of the Ganges to drier upland climates. The ancient Indian elite appear to have accepted this advice with the same enthusiasm as did the English colonial counterparts of the nineteenth and early twentieth centuries.

At the same time, in Europe, a type of establishment, the sanatorium, was developed to treat tuberculosis patients through a therapy based on rest in the open air and a dietary plan. A German doctor named Brehmer (1826–1889) was the first to research the geographical and meteorological conditions favorable to patients, and he observed that mountain regions were relatively spared from the disease, which he explained was due to altitude reducing the atmospheric pressure: an erroneous argument, but significant for medical knowledge of the time. Thereafter, "The therapeutic value of the high altitude climate was not discredited by the evidence of the contagiousness and then the bacterial cause of phthisis: the vague notion of climatic immunity was skillfully converted into a bacteriological asepsis that seemed specific to isolated places – high seas or mountains, for example" (Grandvoinnet 2010). This was enough to convince doctors, such as Paul Jacoby, in 1888, of the therapeutic value of a stay at altitude: "The phthisic will abandon his affairs and leave the city. He will choose a very bare, sterile, cold, windy, sunny plateau nearby, the wind and the sun being excellent disinfectants. In this way, he will place himself more or less in the conditions of a stay in a country of immunity" (Grandvoinnet 2010).

It was therefore a question of proposing places welcoming patients and offering good air, sunshine and a position sheltered from the winds. A form of medical

3 However, attributed to divine wrath.

tourism[4] was developing in sanatoriums with a landscape and architectural impact, which Lüthi (2012) called "an architecture to heal". This meant considering architecture as curative, and care buildings would, therefore, obey principles such as the grouping of patients as close as possible to the doctor and applying hygiene principles previously mentioned, such as promoting the circulation of air and light, all combined with a hotel function. High-altitude destinations, such as Davos or Leysin in Switzerland, became places of treatment, and even after it was discovered that altitude was not the only determinant of healing, the success of these locations as "health destinations" continued. Hospitals everywhere were built according to the precepts of the sanatorium until the 1940s, when they became obsolete with the advent of modern operating theaters. Sanatoriums disappeared after the discovery of streptomycin (an anti-tuberculosis antibiotic), which made these buildings and treatment stays redundant. Nevertheless, the increase in the number of cases of resistance to antibiotics that is currently observed could one day lead to a loss of effectiveness of these treatments and we would then see the sanatoriums come back into service.

Beyond climate, nature is considered to have health-promoting virtues. The concept underlying this vision is that of ecosystem health, which comprises aspects which may be either positive (health benefits of visiting protected natural spaces) or negative (negative effects on human health due to the degradation of the natural environment, water and air pollution, degradation of wetlands, and so on).

This approach still persists today. Thus, the Ottawa Charter (WHO 1986) points out that protection of the environment and natural resources are essential elements in any health promotion strategy. Scientific literature also contains a large number of studies that highlight, for example, the benefits of visiting natural parks (Bowler et al. 2010). These studies describe the short-term benefits of physical activity in parks, public gardens and green spaces (some may object that it is the benefits of the activity itself on health, and not those of nature, that are measured here). The studies also describe the benefits to mental health, particularly through the use of self-reported well-being emotion indicators, which improve with more frequent visits to natural spaces. Other studies have attempted to statistically relate this frequentation to physiological indicators, such as blood pressure or cortisol (a hormone linked to cholesterol) levels, but the results are less conclusive.

Modern Western societies have become accustomed to using green spaces in their daily leisure activities to offer themselves a little "nature" in the middle of urban spaces and during tourist stays, such as in national parks. A study published in

4 The topic of medical tourism is developed in Chapter 3 of this book.

2015 (Romagosa et al. 2015) explores the role of parks and nature conservation areas as contributors to human health and well-being. Natural protected areas allow the preservation of healthy environments and resources necessary for health (such as drinking water or unpolluted land); they can constitute ethnobotanical reservoirs for pharmacopoeia or simply constitute privileged observatories, useful in botany and applied to health. Finally, they constitute places conducive to physical exercise and therapeutic activities (such as convalescence). Five contributions of parks and natural areas to health and well-being have been identified: physical, mental, spiritual, social and environmental (Maller et al. 2008). In detail, these contributions have very concrete translations: the following are a few random examples by way of illustration. Visiting parks and protected natural areas allows for better post-operative recovery, better control of blood pressure, obesity or osteoporosis; it can reinforce healthy consumption habits through the promotion of local products and brands associated with these protected areas; it allows visitors to immerse themselves in landscapes that can have therapeutic virtues (Gesler 1992) and contribute to better mental health, for example, through physical activity that involves setting a goal and surpassing ourselves in order to achieve it, thus reinforcing self-esteem; finally, nature is a space for intergenerational meetings that is favorable for the social dimension of health.

The invention of national parks and outdoor recreation were the results of an interest in the protection of nature (Richez 1992), and are the precursors of another dimension that today links tourism, sustainable development and health through the dimensions of physical activity and resourcing. "The interest is as much in how experience within the landscape [and nature] can act as a prophylaxis against illness as in how it may moderate causes or mitigate effects of ill-health, mental or physical" (Thompson 2011). For this same author, frequenting natural spaces is conducive to psychological balance, and notions such as active and picturesque curiosity or mental pleasure, derived from contemplating the beauties of nature, prefigure certain theories of modern psychology.

Thus, while Thompson argues very strongly around the idea of the health benefits of getting out of the city for activities in nature, this nature can itself be brought into the city, in the form of parks where leisure activities can be practiced and provide health benefits.

In summary, from ancient practices, a process of democratization of tourism was initiated and a relationship between tourism and health was built around practices (baths and treatments) that were linked to medicine to a greater or lesser extent, according to the times, and around environmental issues (nature protection) linked to hedonistic, aesthetic and well-being dimensions.

1.4. From heliotropism to a reflection on social inequalities in tourism

The development of tourism linked to health and well-being occurred in the wealthy societies of the west and, before the democratization of paid vacations in the 1930s, was even reserved for an aristocratic elite. While a large proportion of the population of Westernized countries has access to tourism today, enormous imbalances and inequalities continue between rich and poor countries. Inequalities in health (social and territorial) are, however, a major theme in health research and particularly in the social sciences of health. It is therefore logical and relevant to raise this question of inequalities through the prism of the relationship between tourism and health. It is also clear that there has been very little work done in this field. However, since the 1980s, authors such as G. Cazes have studied the changes in developing nations due to the effect of tourism practices based on a structural imbalance between, on the one hand, a tourist industry based on the pursuit of pleasure and, on the other hand, local communities whose scarce resources are taken over. The development of globalized tourism is based on heliotropism (the development of sun tourism, which involves taking a sun cure in countries that are mostly the result of colonization (such as Tunisia, Morocco and Senegal for France) by taking advantage of a difference in living standards that allows for low-cost stays based on infrastructures and practices inherited from colonialism (Boukhri and Chapuis 2016).

In a book entitled *Curing the Colonizers*, Jennings studies the history of thermalism and climatism[5] in the French colonial empire: “As early as the 19th century, thermalism combined with climatism appeared to be a way to arrest the high mortality rates in hot countries, but also to ‘recharge’ colonials either through thermal cures in the Madagascan, Reunionese, West Indian and Tunisian ‘Vichys’, or by repatriating the colonials towards metropolitan spa towns.” The aim was, to a certain extent, to recreate a little piece of Europe in the colonies (Figure 1.11). According to Boukhris and Chapuis, the resorts created at the time were “planned at altitude or by the sea in order to seek the freshness and mildness of a more temperate climate”, in order to encourage the rest of the colonists as well as certain hedonistic practices, notably forms of sexual tourism. Tourism thus solidified the colonial power in these places and produced “exotic imaginaries” that are still at work today in the promotion of tourist destinations.

5 Author’s note: search for a healthy climate with regard to a pathology.

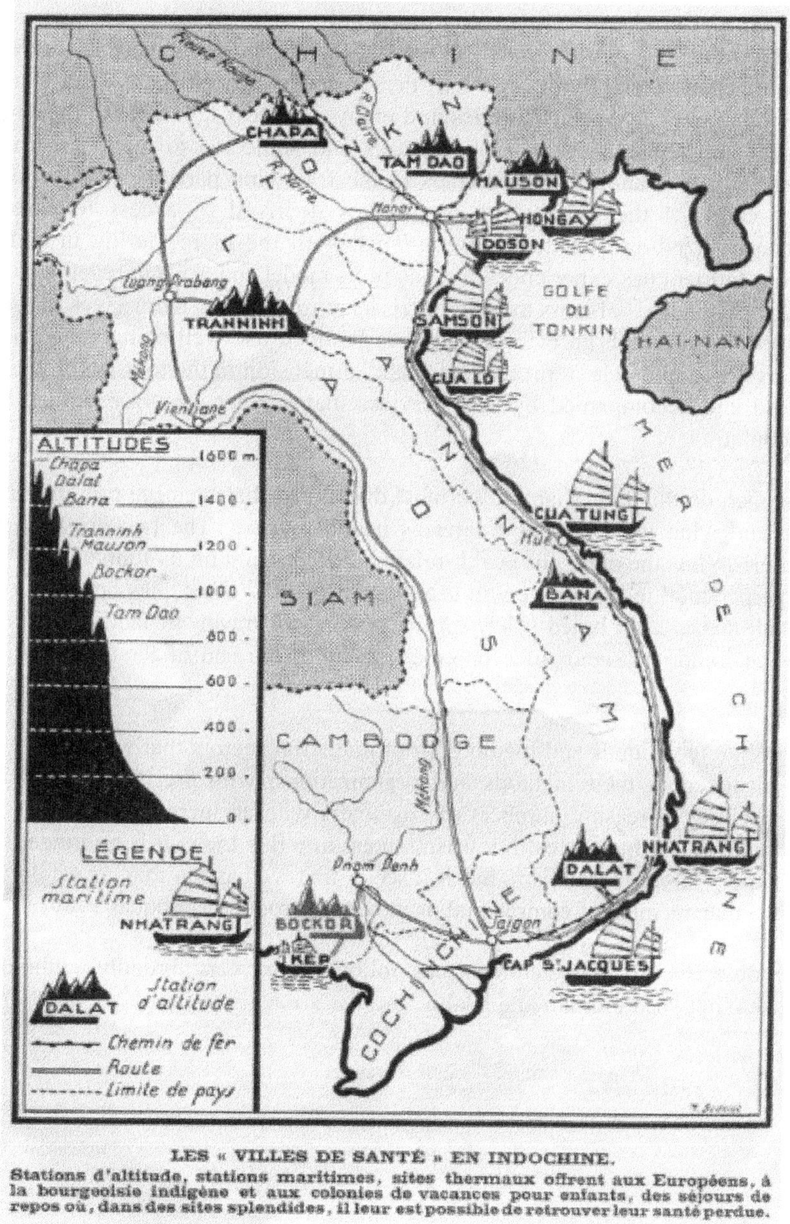

Figure 1.11. *Reproduction of the figure of the climate stations in Indochina (source: Le Monde colonial illustré, no. 180, 1938)*

These spaces produced during colonization have remained highly unequal, and the gap between the society of tourists and the society that operates these leisure spaces is immense, particularly with regard to their respective health and quality of life. Tourists relax, recharge their batteries and enjoy a context favorable to their health, while staff are kept busy with arduous tasks and subjected to work patterns that are often harmful[6], and all of this leads to the following paradox: staff who have to "take care" of the tourists are themselves deprived of access to care in a compartmentalized and unequal system. This is all the more glaring in countries where sun tourism has experienced a crisis in its model and is being redefined. These hedonistic destinations of mass tourism in crisis are reinventing themselves in order to target new sectors with an offer of services branded as "well-being" and "health" and a privileged clientele: retirees. The "care" dimension in the tourism offer is thus reinforced and accompanied by new services that are not always extended to the local population.

To conclude this first chapter, we must distinguish between the role of health in tourism and what we will define later as health tourism. The two are linked, but while tourism has the quest for health-related wellness among its foundations, which is still perpetuated today, as we will see, there are many other links between tourism and health that are not based solely on the reasons for travel. In fact, when tourism became an important sector of economic activity at the end of the 20th century, it had to

> utilize techniques and methods from industrial sectors that were more advanced in their methods and organizations, with the objective of reaching increasing numbers of customers with an increasingly broad range of products. Health tourism enters into this logic. It is no longer simply about thermalism, but is a sector that we have to treat as we do the management of commercial or industrial products (Lanquar 1989)

The objective of the chapters that follow is to very broadly embrace the relationship between tourism and health.

---

6 This point is developed in Chapter 4 of this book.

2

Travel Health, Risks and Diseases

At the beginning of 2020, the world watched in shock at the rapid spread of a virus from China, SARS-CoV-2, otherwise known as Covid-19. This virus appeared in the Wuhan region of China and spread worldwide via air transport, demonstrating how planet Earth now functions as a vast interconnected system. International tourist mobility and business mobility are clearly part of this system. The flows and profiles of travelers are well documented, and there is a body of literature that informs us about the main health risks and morbidity associated with travel. Covid-19 will of course be discussed in this chapter and like Rial (2020) we will ask "how will we travel after the pandemic?" However, let us not lose sight of the fact that it was known long before the coronavirus crisis that travel-related morbidity is largely dominated by communicable diseases (Le Bras et al. 1992; Bouchaud 2003). The SARS-CoV-2 pandemic should therefore not obscure other health problems that may affect the traveling tourist.

> The proportion of travelers complaining of any kind of health problem is around 60%, with variations of between 15 and 78% depending on the study, and the famous diarrhea, or turista, affects nearly one in two travelers. On the other hand, some typically tropical diseases particularly feared by travelers, are relatively, or even very rare: 2 to 3% for malaria, 3 in 100,000 for typhoid fever and 3 in 1,000,000 for cholera. Some much less 'exotic' health problems are more frequent and often serious: 1 in 3 medical repatriations result from trauma, 1 in 3 from cardiovascular events and nearly 1 in 10 from psychiatric collapse. (Bouchaud 2003)

For a color version of all the figures in this chapter, see: www.iste.co.uk/fleuret/tourism.zip.

Before even considering how diseases and their infectious agents can travel, it is useful to understand the main areas of distribution of diseases across the globe and, from there, to identify the main areas at risk. The areas thus identified must then be compared with tourist areas and activities.

2.1. Diseases and risk areas

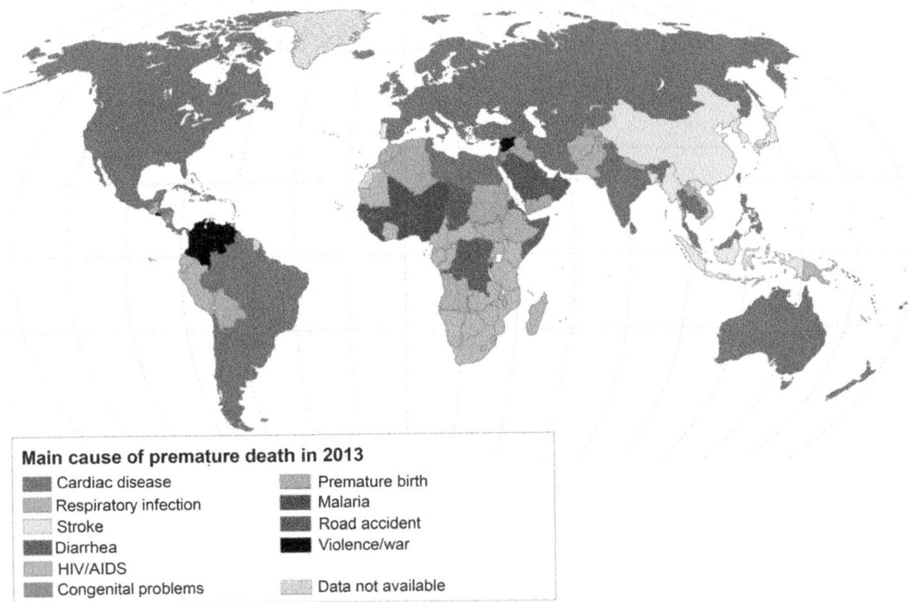

Figure 2.1. *Primary causes of premature mortality by country (source: GBD 2013; Mortality and Causes of Death Collaborators, Global, regional and national age-sex specific all-cause and cause-specific mortality for 240 causes of death, 1990–2013, The Lancet, 2014; background map: FNSP. Sciences Po – Cartography workshop CC BY 4.0; design and production: Fleuret S., Lepetit A., UMR 6590 ESO)*

The main causes of mortality vary considerably depending on the country (Figure 2.1), in connection with a phenomenon known as the epidemiological, or health transition. This transition occurs when a country experiences a significant improvement in hygiene, nutrition and health services, which is what happened in western countries in connection with the Industrial Revolution. There then followed a decrease in infant mortality and a progressive increase in life expectancy. Over the course of history, different countries around the world have entered into this epidemiological transition at different rates and some have not yet achieved it. This transition has resulted in a transformation in the causes of death: the infectious diseases that dominated before the transition are gradually losing their significance, while the proportion of chronic and degenerative diseases and accidents in the causes of death is increasing.

As can be seen in Figure 2.1, a north-south divide exists, although it is tending to fade in places. There are still areas of high prevalence of infectious and parasitic diseases and this is a specific issue for tourism, which brings populations from areas where the "culture" of infectious disease and certain natural protections through the development of antibodies may have been lost to risk zones (Le Bras et al. 1992). Gautret et al. (2009) have shown that depending on their origin, people do not all contract exactly the same diseases when traveling.

Travel medicine is a discipline that focuses specifically on the health risks associated with international mobility, using a biomedical approach. The development of this discipline "has made it possible to improve the prevention of diseases contracted during international travel and their detection upon return from such travel, whether for tourists or migrants" (Rey 2007). However, this approach does not systematically integrate the social and cultural parameters usually dealt with in the human and social sciences. Thus, to paraphrase Maximilien Sorre, the biological foundations of the geography of tourism remain to be written.

2.1.1. *Infectious and parasitic diseases*

Infectious and parasitic diseases are caused by viruses (examples include: AIDS, measles, influenza and SARS) or by bacteria (pneumonia, tuberculosis, diphtheria and so on), in the case of infectious diseases, and by parasites (ascariasis, filariasis, amebiasis, malaria and so on) in the case of parasitic diseases. Some microscopic fungi can also cause infectious diseases.

These diseases can be transmitted, directly or indirectly, from person to person. Zoonotic diseases are infectious diseases, the reservoir of which is found in animals, and which can be transmitted to humans.

The impact of infectious and parasitic diseases shows a very high geographical variability, with the African continent being by far the worst affected (Figure 2.2).

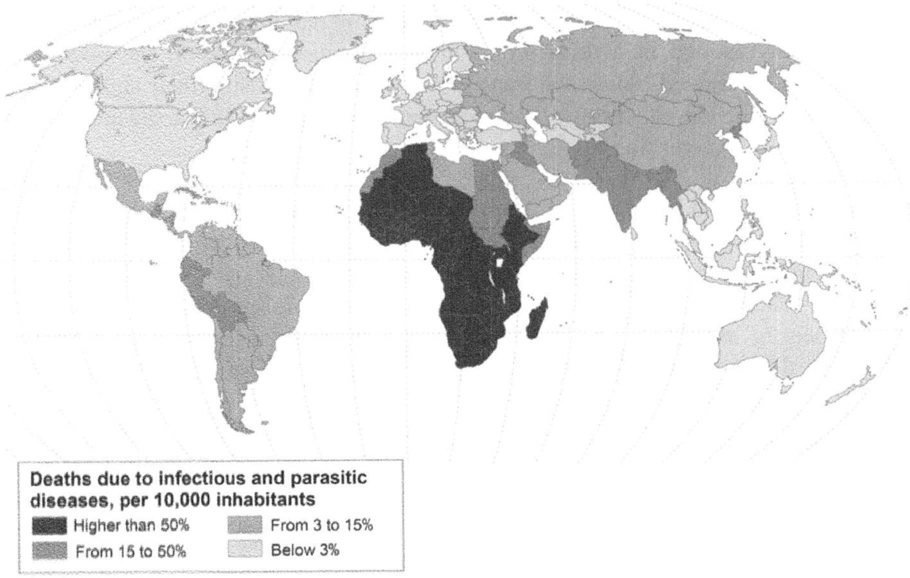

Figure 2.2. *Worldwide deaths from infectious and parasitic diseases (source: World Health Organization, 2016; UNDP – World Bank Institut Pasteur; background map: FNSP. Sciences Po – Cartography workshop CC BY 4.0; production: Lepetit A., UMR 6590 ESO)*

The aim here is not to draw up a complete inventory of infectious and parasitic diseases that may interact with tourists, either by infecting them or by being spread by them. Instead, we will restrict ourselves to a broad outline of the main infections that tourists and tourism professionals should keep in mind for the potential risks they represent. We will discuss vector-borne diseases, orofecal infections (which will lead us to discuss hygiene-related risks), parasites and finally sexually transmitted diseases.

2.1.1.1. *Vector-borne diseases*

Vectors are organisms (primarily blood-sucking insects and mites) that transmit pathogens or parasites from one infected individual (or animal) to another, thus causing serious disease in human populations. They are generally found in tropical and subtropical regions and where access to clean water and sanitation systems is a problem.

Globally, it is estimated that vector-borne diseases account for around 17% of infectious diseases. Malaria, a disease transmitted by mosquitoes, is the disease that has claimed the most victims (estimated at 228 million in 2018, according to the WHO), with several hundred thousand deaths each year, although mortality is declining (660,000 deaths in 2010, down to 405,000 in 2018, again according to the WHO).

While the number of deaths from malaria is decreasing, there is one vector-borne disease that is spreading very rapidly in the world: dengue. Its incidence has increased 30-fold in the last 50 years.

International tourism can be a vector for the spread of these diseases. Each year, approximately 50 million people travel from industrialized to tropical countries, which are the main sources of vector-borne diseases. In so doing, they expose themselves to various diseases, particularly through insect bites (these are known as arboviruses). Mosquitoes are the principal vectors of many pathogens responsible for human diseases, such as malaria, dengue, chikungunya and yellow fever.

Malaria is a disease caused by a parasite, *Plasmodium*, which is transmitted by female *Anopheles* mosquitoes that carry it. In humans, these parasites multiply in the liver and then attack red blood cells. There are five types of these parasites, but two are particularly dangerous: *P. falciparum*, which is found in Africa, Southeast Asia, the eastern Mediterranean and the Pacific; and *P. vivax*, which is found in the Americas. Malaria manifests itself through high fevers that, if not promptly treated, can progress to severe and often fatal disease. There is no truly effective vaccine at this time; the disease is treated with artemisinin-based combination therapy (ACT). According to Mouchet et al. (1993),

> faced with the aggression of parasites and, in particular, of *P. falciparum*, subjects living in endemic areas develop defenses that are all the more solid and precocious, as they are regularly subjected to the infecting Anopheles bites. This premunition, an armed peace between the parasite and its host, translates into the presence of a very high number of carriers, who present no clinical signs, in regions of high transmission. It is established at the cost of a high rate of infant and child mortality, but afterwards, adults more or less escape the pathological effects of malaria.

The malaria zones are well known (Figure 2.3). According to the WHO, the geographical areas where transmission is most intense are those where mosquitoes live long enough for the parasite to complete its development cycle inside them, which explains why around 90% of malaria cases worldwide occur in Africa (where mosquitoes prefer to bite humans rather than animals). Transmission is also affected by climatic conditions that determine the abundance and life span of mosquitoes. In some parts of the world, seasonal peaks in transmission are observed during or just after the rainy season. Malaria epidemics can occur when climate and other conditions suddenly favor transmission in areas where populations have little or no immunity. They can also occur when people with low immunity move to areas of high transmission, to find work, for example, or as refugees. In these areas, the tourist is also an intruder who is merely passing through without being protected against the disease, but the limited duration of the stay means that the risk of infection remains individual and not epidemic. Nevertheless, prophylaxis[1] (taking preventive medication) is essential for these visitors as well as the use of mosquito nets and repellents. Too many establishments welcoming tourists still lack this basic protection. Moreover, it is formally advised that pregnant women and young children should not travel to malaria zones unless there are compelling reasons, of which tourism is not one!

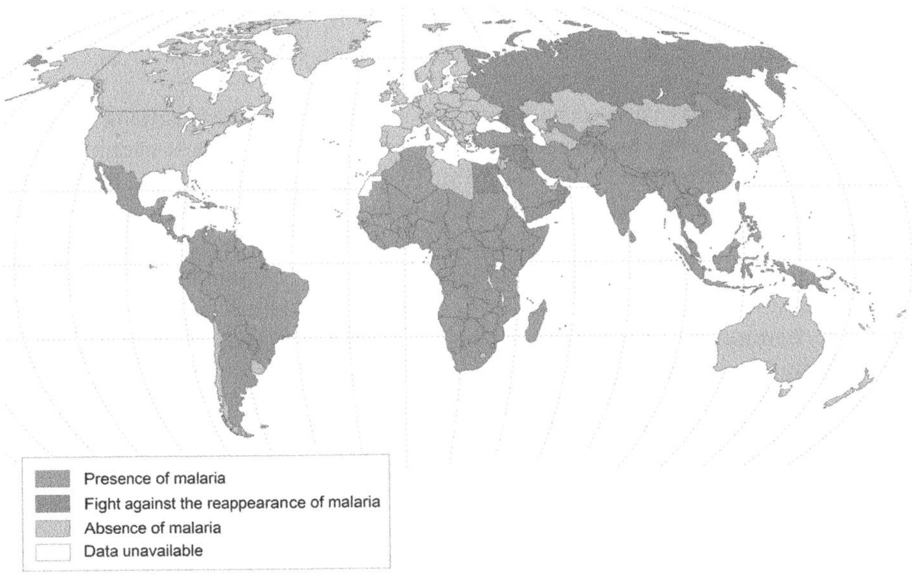

Figure 2.3. *World malaria zones (source: World Health Organization, 2012; background map: FNSP. Sciences Po – Cartography workshop CC BY 4.0; production: Lepetit A., UMR 6590 ESO)*

Less widespread than malaria, but made famous by a recent epidemic, chikungunya is a so-called "emerging" viral disease that causes fever and severe joint

1 We will not develop the subject of medication here, but due to the numerous resistances that have appeared to certain treatments, tourists who visit a malaria zone must seek competent medical advice before their stay, especially since prescriptions vary according to the destination (and the level of resistance to chloroquine that is observed there), as well as according to the sensitivity of each individual to the side effects of treatments, which can be serious.

pain. Also known as "the chik" or the "bent man" disease (Taglioni 2010), it can affect any population without effective curative treatment. Only analgesics and anti-inflammatories are prescribed in case of attacks, and they only treat the symptoms, not the cause of the disease itself. Prevention is limited to self-protection against mosquito bites, as there is no vaccine against this disease. Beyond the health consequences of an epidemic, there are many political, economic and social consequences when a virus affects a tourist area, as was the case between 2004 and 2006 in the Indian Ocean, from Reunion Island to Mauritius via the Seychelles and the Comoros, with an observed prevalence of 20–60% of the population, depending on the island (Taglioni 2010). On Reunion Island, nearly 300,000 people were affected under the watchful eye of the media, which relayed this health crisis around the world. Epidemiologically, it is assumed that the virus endemic to east Africa may have traveled initially to the Comoros and then to the Seychelles, Reunion and Mauritius, possibly carried by in-transit tourists within this geographical area. The vector of this disease is the *Aedes albopictus*, or Asian tiger mosquito. While some diseases travel and spread by taking humans as host and vector of contagion (as we will see later), here it is the mosquito that has traveled, which raises the fear that the epidemic may spread to other areas where the tiger mosquito is already present or has favorable conditions in which to establish itself. This is the case, for example, in northern Italy and Provence. However, we know that "85% of the 400,000 tourists on Reunion come from Europe, with an overwhelming proportion from France. In Mauritius, two thirds of the 900,000 tourists who visit the island are European, with French nationals accounting for 25% of the annual total, and, in the Seychelles, a majority (80%) of the 160,000 annual tourists are European" (Taglioni 2010). The risk is therefore that chikungunya vector mosquitoes are traveling in their luggage, etc. In metropolitan France, there were 896 cases of chikungunya concomitant with the epidemic in Reunion. Fortunately, no indigenous cases have been identified. This health crisis has had the effect of raising awareness and reactivating preventive measures, such as the elimination of breeding grounds for the tiger mosquito (hoteliers have a major role to play, for example, in the management of their green spaces and their watering)[2]. Another consequence of this epidemic has been its impact on the economy. A study conducted on Reunion Island showed a drop in turnover of 20–80% reported by hotel establishments during the crisis, with three hotels even being forced to temporarily close due to a lack of customers (Iedom 2006). Tourists flee very quickly from areas affected by a health crisis, especially when that crisis is reported by the media. Another economic and social consequence is linked to the spread of the disease among employees in the tourism sector, where nearly 20% of staff were recorded as being off sick at the height of the crisis.

2 This tendency of western societies, which have long since benefitted as a result of epidemiological transition, to drop their mistrust of infectious and vector-borne diseases would have other consequences during the Covid-19 crisis in 2020, which we will discuss later.

Dengue, also called "tropical flu", is another viral disease carried by mosquitoes (*Aedes aegypti*). It affects infants, young children and adults alike, causing sudden, high fevers. Its hemorrhagic form causes potentially fatal complications, and the WHO estimates that there are 50 million cases annually, including 500,000 cases of dengue hemorrhagic fever, which is fatal in more than 2.5% of cases. Like chikungunya, the dengue vector is likely to establish itself in western countries. *A. aegypti* is already present in 18 French departments and dengue could spread there if infected people arrive uncontrolled in these territories (source: Institut Pasteur 2014). To date, there is neither a specific treatment nor a systematically effective vaccine against this disease. Therefore, the only existing means of control are individual protection against mosquito bites (repellents and wearing long clothing) and control of mosquito vectors. This means, for example, spraying insecticides on international flights from infested areas, which may raise further questions about the harmfulness of the products used.

Moreover, this may well prove to be totally inadequate. An early study (1987, cited by Rodriguez-Garcia (2001)) involved placing mosquitoes in the landing gear of a Boeing 747. After approximately 24 hours in the air, the plane arrived at its destination and the mosquitoes were checked: they were all alive and "doing well".

Yellow fever is the third major viral disease transmitted by the bite of *Aedes* mosquitoes and can cause devastating outbreaks in the tropical regions of Africa and Central and South America. In addition to fever, the most common symptoms of yellow fever are myalgia (especially back pain), headache, loss of appetite, nausea and vomiting. In most cases, the symptoms disappear after three or four days. In a small number of cases, a higher fever returns after a short remission and several organs are affected, such as the liver and kidneys, causing jaundice (yellowing of the skin and eyes, hence the name "yellow fever"). Half of the patients with this toxic phase die within seven to ten days. It is therefore a very serious disease, but, unlike the two diseases described above, it is possible to avoid these epidemics because a vaccine exists, which is inexpensive, effective and safe. A mass vaccination campaign gives protection to 99% of those vaccinated after 30 days. Tourists should, of course, be vaccinated before traveling to an endemic area. Some countries require a vaccination certificate before entry into their territory. An Eliminate Yellow fever Epidemics (EYE) strategy was launched in 2017 in 40 at-risk countries in Africa and the Americas. The goal is that, by 2026, more than 1 billion people will be protected from the disease.

Japanese encephalitis is another viral disease whose vector is the mosquito. Although relatively rare (less than 70,000 cases recorded per year), its acute form has a case fatality rate of nearly 30%, and, of those who survive, 30–50% have permanent neurological or psychiatric aftereffects. It is endemic to 24 countries in Southeast Asia and the western Pacific and is manifested by fever and headaches. In its acute form (about 1 in 250 cases), it results in the sudden onset of high fever, headaches, stiff neck, disorientation, coma, convulsions, spastic paralysis and death (source: WHO). There is no cure, but a safe and effective vaccine is available.

There are other lesser known but equally serious vector-borne diseases.

Crimean–Congo hemorrhagic fever is a disease caused by a virus transmitted by ticks and livestock (which can be infected by a tick bite). The disease causes outbreaks of severe viral hemorrhagic fever. It is endemic in Africa, the Balkans, the Middle East and Asia, but the geographical limit north of which the vector is no longer found is 50 degrees northern latitude. Human-to-human transmission is possible but involves direct contact with blood, secretion, organs or body fluids of infected individuals. Hence, it is important that any tourist who falls ill after a trip informs the healthcare personnel who is taking care of them of the geographical areas they have visited and any bites they may have contracted (in this case, a tick bite), which may put the healthcare personnel on alert.

Lymphatic filariasis is caused by a parasite inoculated by mosquitoes: a nematode-like worm of the filaridae family, hence the name of the disease. It causes an alteration of the lymphatic system (which participates in the detoxification of organs and the body and allows the circulation of white blood cells in the body – outside the blood vessels – thus contributing to the immune system). Lymphatic filariasis can also cause hypertrophy of certain parts of the body, which is why it is often called elephantiasis (which has nothing to do with the case of the Elephant Man, John Merrick, who was, in fact, suffering from a genetic disease).

Chagas disease is a potentially fatal disease caused by a protozoan, *Trypanosoma cruzi*. It is estimated that 6–7 million people have contracted this disease, mainly in an endemic area comprising 21 Latin American countries. With Chagas disease, the bite of the vector introduces a parasite into the human body that multiplies in the acute phase of the disease (which is relatively asymptomatic, but then the disease becomes chronic when the parasite lodges in the heart muscle and in the digestive muscles, causing lesions). It is not a contagious disease, and, according to the WHO, is transmitted to humans mainly via

> triatomine bugs (a type of bedbug) that generally live in cracks in walls of precarious dwellings in rural or suburban areas. These triatomine bugs hide during the day and come out at night to feed on

mammal blood, including that of humans. They bite an exposed area of skin, such as the face, and defecate or urinate near the bite. The parasites enter the body when the person instinctively rubs or scratches and cause the droppings to enter the lesion, eyes, mouth, or other skin alteration.

Bilharzia, or schistosomiasis, is a disease caused by parasites released into the water by gastropods. The risk of infection is linked to contact with infested water during agricultural, domestic or leisure activities (such as swimming). Schistosomiasis particularly affects poor communities that do not have access to safe drinking water and satisfactory sanitation in subtropical and tropical regions (92% of patients are in Africa). However, with the development of ecotourism and off-the-beaten-track travel, an increasing number of tourists are contracting schistosomiasis. With regard to symptoms, these can be localized in different parts of the body and cause abdominal pain, diarrhea and the appearance of blood in stools, when it is intestinal, and in urine when it is urogenital. It is a chronic disease that disables more than it kills, but can have serious long-term consequences.

Leptospirosis is found throughout the world. The main reservoirs of this bacterial disease are rodents, especially rats, which excrete bacteria in their urine and thus contaminate the environment (fresh water, muddy soils). Animal farms and their effluents can also be reservoirs of contamination. In humans, the disease is often benign, but can lead to renal failure, or even death in severe forms, which are estimated at one million per year worldwide, according to the Institut Pasteur. In its moderate form, the disease resembles flu-like symptoms. It may progress to cause renal, hepatic, meningeal or pulmonary attacks, and, in 20% of cases, it is complicated by a hemorrhagic syndrome. Convalescence is long, but generally without aftereffects. People who practice water sports (such as swimming, canoeing, kayaking, fishing, hunting and canyoning) are considered more at risk. Bacteria can contaminate them by penetrating mainly through skin wounds or mucous membranes.

African trypanosomiasis, also known as sleeping sickness, is a widespread tropical disease that can be fatal if untreated, and is transmitted by the bite of the notorious tsetse fly. It is found exclusively in sub-Saharan Africa (36 countries are affected) and, thanks to active control programs, the number of cases is steadily decreasing: 2009 saw the number fall below 10,000 and in 2018 only 977 new cases were reported. Nevertheless, efforts must be maintained. The disease had indeed already strongly regressed in the 1960s when it seemed under control at around

5,000 cases per year. However, after a slackening of vigilance, there was a resurgence in the disease and it again caused many tens of thousands of cases per year. In the first phase, sleeping sickness is relatively asymptomatic and therefore difficult to detect. The initial symptoms are fever, pain, joint pain and pruritus. The disease then reaches the central nervous system and can become fatal. Although sleeping sickness can be treated, its diagnosis and treatment are complex, but the earlier the diagnosis, the better the prospects for recovery.

The list of vector-borne diseases is long and multifaceted and is responsible for many deaths worldwide (Figure 2.4), but we will call a halt to our inventory there, pointing out that the fight against these diseases relies at least as much on prevention and sanitation of risk environments as it does on care. The same is true for the group of water-related diseases presented below (which also includes parasitic diseases).

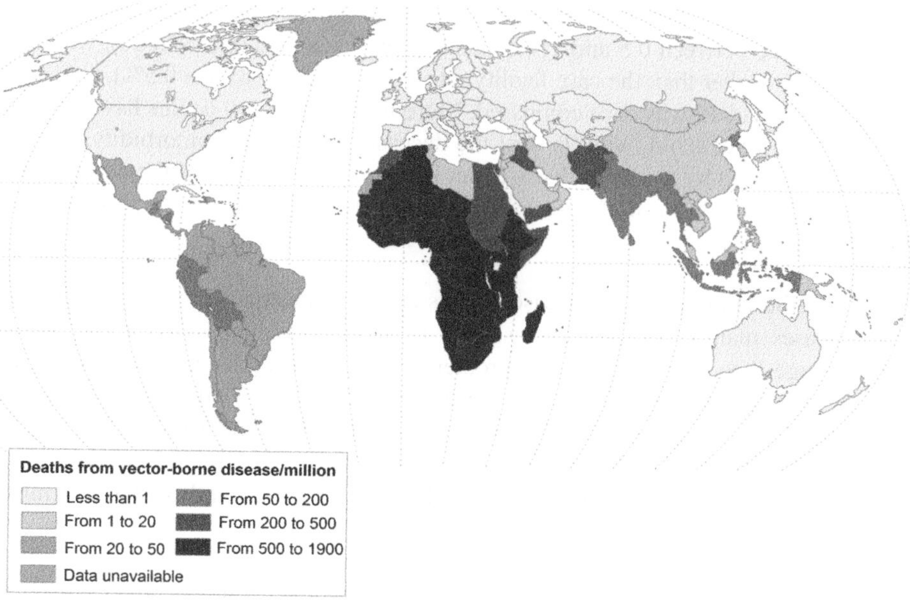

Figure 2.4. *Worldwide deaths due to vector-borne diseases (source: World Health Organization, 2004; background map: FNSP. Sciences Po – Cartography workshop CC BY 4.0; design and production: Fleuret S., Lepetit A., UMR 6590 ESO)*

2.1.1.2. *The very special case of Covid-19*

The disease caused by the coronavirus SARS-CoV-2, or Covid-19, is an infectious, zoonotic and emerging disease. Although its origins are not precisely known, the greatest likelihood is that it is a virus that had a bat as its host and mutated to be transmissible to humans in a process yet to be ascertained. The first cases appeared at the end of 2019 in the Wuhan region in China, and, in a few weeks, Covid-19 became a global pandemic. The particularity of this disease, of which little is understood, is that it is, in a large number of cases, asymptomatic and therefore undetectable. In other cases, it results in an infection of the respiratory tract, flu-like symptoms and sometimes a loss of taste and smell. It is a relatively contagious virus that is transmitted between humans and can spread very rapidly. It is fatal in a limited number of cases, but its case fatality rate is particularly complicated to calculate since the exact number of infected people is not known due to the many asymptomatic cases that have gone undetected (especially since diagnosis requires a PCR test[3], which was not available at the beginning of the pandemic). This rate is estimated to be between 0.5 and 1% depending on the source (OMS 2020), which is clearly much higher than the case fatality rate of influenza (less than 0.5%), a disease with which Covid-19 was once compared. More than 8 out of 10 deaths have been in people over 75 years old, with 95% of the deceased presenting comorbidity, that is, they were affected by a serious disease that increased the severity of the coronavirus infection. Finally, 76% of the deceased suffered from cardiovascular disease and 40% had diabetes.

This is therefore a serious disease, but its lethality remains relatively low and its serious cases mainly (but not exclusively) concern populations with a risk factor related to age or to pre-existing health problems. Its seriousness is in its rate of spread and in the existence of severe forms of respiratory infections requiring hospitalization and even, in many cases, a stay in intensive care. The high number of these severe cases, and their occurrence over a very short period of time, has contributed to a saturation of hospital capacities, putting the health systems of most countries in the world at risk.

Since the end of 2020, several vaccines have become available, suggesting that the crisis may be resolved in the medium term. However, before a collective immunity is reached (which remains uncertain to this day because of the need for a booster dose), it will have been necessary to go through phases of strict lockdown.

3 Polymerase Chain Reaction, a molecular biology technique for in vitro gene amplification.

The first of these was declared in Wuhan on January 23, 2020. An incredulous world watched as the city's 12 million inhabitants were placed in quarantine, and yet, as we would later learn, the virus was already circulating outside China by this date. Figure 2.5 illustrates the speed with which the disease spread and became a global pandemic through one very telling indicator: the lockdown measures decreed by each country. This figure also shows that the impact of these measures has been long-lasting, with major social and economic consequences, and obviously tourism has been affected, both nationally and internationally. Indeed, many countries took measures to close their borders in order to limit the circulation of the virus. International transport was particularly affected and virtually brought to a halt by the paralysis of international air traffic from March 2020, as shown in Figure 2.6.

According to the UNWTO, in 2020, "destinations welcomed 900 million fewer international tourists between January and October, compared with the same period in 2019". Again according to the UNWTO, this was the "worst year in the history of the tourism sector". The whole world has been affected, which is reflected, for example, in the numbers of tourist arrivals. In Asia and the Pacific, the first regions to be affected by the pandemic and where travel restrictions have been most severe, there was an 82% decrease in arrivals in the first ten months of 2020. The Middle East saw a 73% decline, and Africa 69%. International arrivals to Europe and the Americas decreased by 68% (source: UNWTO World Tourism Barometer, December 2020).

Ultimately, the SARS-CoV-2 coronavirus will have had a major impact on the tourism sector, not only by preventing tourists from traveling, but also by causing the closure of the most emblematic sites and attractions, the cancellation or postponement of many festivals and cultural events, and by making it necessary to ban public gatherings (indoor and outdoor) in many countries as part of social distancing measures designed to curb the spread of the virus. Moreover, according to the OECD (2020), "the magnitude and depth of the Covid-19-related effects on tourism and the economy in general make a rapid recovery unlikely".

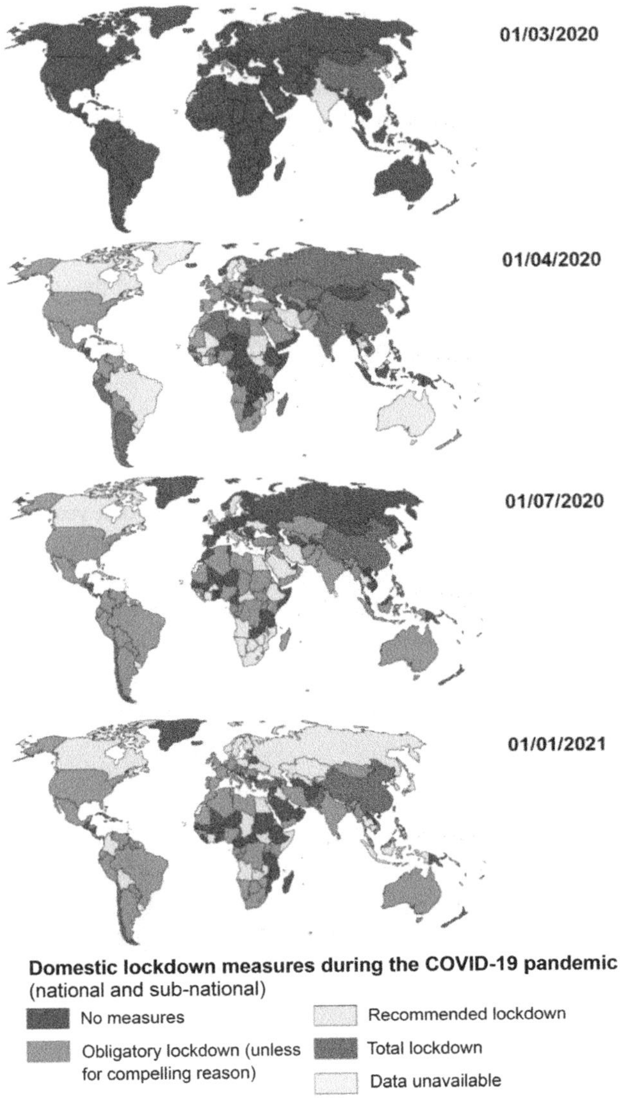

Figure 2.5. *Spread of lockdown measures during the Covid-19 pandemic (source: Hale, Agrist, Goldszmidt, Kira, Petherick, Philips, Webster, Cameron-Blake, Hallas, Majumdar and Tatlow 2021, "A global panel database of pandemic policies (Oxford Covid-19 Government Response Tracker)", Nature Human Behavior, https://ourworldindata.org/coronavirus)*

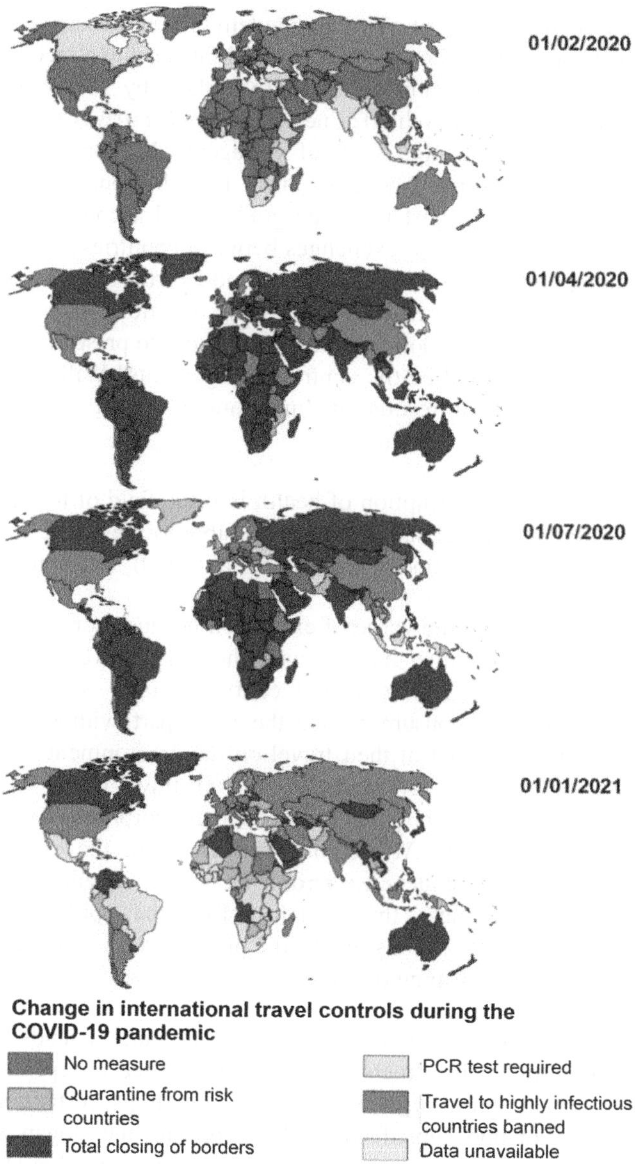

Figure 2.6. *International air traffic shutdown during the Covid-19 pandemic (source: Hale, Agrist, Goldszmidt, Kira, Petherick, Philips, Webster, Cameron-Blake, Hallas, Majumdar and Tatlow, 2021, "A global panel database of pandemic policies (Oxford COVID-19 Government Response Tracker)", Nature Human Behavior, https://ourworldindata.org/coronavirus)*

If we consider the probability of a similar pandemic event occurring in the future, we must learn the lessons of the Covid-19 crisis. Will this lead to a reconsideration of the tourism model? This question is explicitly asked by the World Tourism Organization in the title of its March 2021 newsletter: *This crisis is an opportunity to rethink the tourism sector*[4]. J.-F. Rial, CEO of Voyageurs du Monde, made a similar point in April 2020 for the Terra Nova think tank[5]. First, he considered scenarios for the end of the crisis. This will most likely be gradual and accompanied by control measures (such as limiting travel to exchanges between countries where the virus is no longer circulating and introducing a health passport certifying that the traveler is immune). These precautionary measures raise many questions: how long will they have to be implemented (e.g. how long will it be mandatory to present a negative PCR test in order to fly?)? What will be the control arrangements? Will they be fair and not liberticidal? Will tourism resume its internationalization or will we see a long-term increase in domestic tourism?

Finally, and above all, this irruption of health into the field of tourism raises the question of a before and after crisis: will it be possible in the future to think about tourism again without thinking about health? For Rial (2020), we should not dream:

> Mass tourism is not on the verge of extinction because consumers are in favor of it. On the other hand, those who today travel in a more responsible and ecological way will continue to do so. Globally, travelers will remain consumers, for the most part without serious concerns about the impact of their travel on the environment. Even if the market shrinks for a few years, changes in travel habits will not come naturally to travelers […] The great metamorphosis for travel will come from politics. While, on the one hand, the crisis will generate nationalistic tendencies across the world, it will also feed the ecological awareness that began before the epidemic. The epidemiological threat remains one of the primary risks mentioned by specialists in global warming or biodiversity.

In spring 2021, the island of Mallorca in the Balearic Islands provided an illustration of this problem. Its streets were almost deserted except for a few rare tourists, mostly German. On a large number of tourist shops, restaurants and bars, and on the balconies of unoccupied hotels, banners with the slogan *SOS turismo* could be seen, while a counter-campaign took up the same graphic style with the slogan *SOS tenible*[6] (Figure 2.7).

4 www.unwto.org/un-tourism-news-21.

5 https://tnova.fr/notes/comment-voyagerons-nous-apres-la-pandemie.

6 *Sostenible* in Spanish can be translated into English as "sustainable".

The *SOS turismo* movement comprises 901 actors and entities from the tourism economy in the Balearic Islands. The manifesto of this movement is explicit:

> In the Balearic Islands, the Covid-19 crisis has caused a drop in GDP of more than 25%. Economic activity is practically paralyzed and is doing little more than surviving. As tourism professionals, we can't hold out much longer.[7]

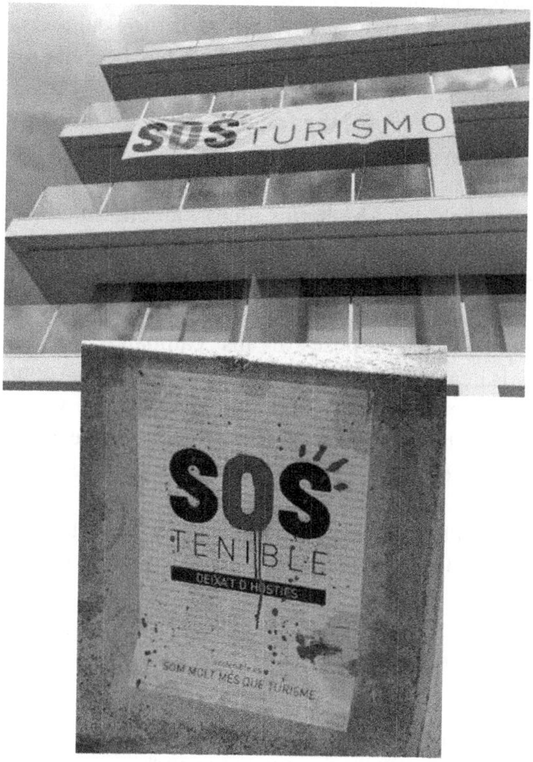

Figure 2.7. *Activist campaigns in reaction to the Covid-19 crisis in the Balearic Islands (photos: S. Fleuret 2021)*

The claims are explicit, the *SOS turismo* movement calls for clearly planned action and priority to measures that would avoid a social crisis, a vaccination policy that would achieve a vaccination rate of 70% for the summer season, a vaccine accreditation system to facilitate international travel for vaccinated tourists and support for businesses, some of which have been closed since October 2019 and

7 https://sosturismo.es/en/, accessed 04/26/2021.

which face insurmountable debts. Consequently, the signatories of this manifesto call for a rescue plan for the tourism sector "the aim of which must be to save businesses and jobs". Finally, *SOS turismo* identifies the issue related to the future return of tourists by calling for a strong message to be sent to countries sending tourists with a view to restoring confidence and showing that work on health security is being undertaken.

Of course, the apparent distress displayed by this protest movement is significant and sincere. Nevertheless, we may ask ourselves if the health crisis is not revealing of a systemic dysfunction. The Balearic archipelago has become totally dependent on tourism, and, what is more, on tourism that is not sufficiently diverse. As a result, the occurrence of a major crisis exposes the fragility of this economy: without tourists, no activity, no income and no solution in sight.

This is the opinion held by Abraham Calero[8], a committed street-art artist living in Mallorca who launched the *SOS tenible* movement, not in opposition to, but in reaction to *SOS turismo*. According to Calero, of course the tourism sector is a key employer in Mallorca, but the solution to the crisis is not a return to the pre-pandemic position. The purpose of his campaign is to criticize the total dependence of the Balearic economy on tourism, which is coupled with negative impacts from overtourism on society and the environment. Calero's objective is to initiate dialogue and use the context of the anticipated crisis recovery as an opportunity to change things and opt for a socially and environmentally sustainable tourism.

In the Balearic Islands, the tourism actors we met all talk about the pre-Covid world and the post-Covid world to come, without knowing what the latter will look like.

2.1.1.3. *Orofecal infections and risks related to water, sanitation and hygiene (WASH)*

Contaminated water, water-contaminated food and dirty hands are the causes of many diseases. We speak of "fecal peril" (CMETE[9]) or orofecal diseases related to the ingestion of contaminated water or food (also called water-borne diseases). These diseases can be of various forms: viral (such as hepatitis and poliomyelitis), bacterial (common diarrhea, typhoid fever, cholera and so on) or digestive parasitic (such as giardiasis and amebiasis). The risk is directly linked to hygiene conditions, access to water and sanitation, and these diseases are common in tropical environments. Tourists are therefore highly exposed in the same way as the local population. They

8 https://www.estilopalma.com/2021/04/abraham-calero-sostenible/, accessed 04/26/2021.

9 Centre médical de médecine du voyage, website: https://www.cmete.com/bilan-de-sante/recommandations-generales-aux-voyageurs/les-maladies-a-transmission-hydrique-et-alimentaire/babArticle_49, accessed 03/20/2020.

are even at the origin of a term used to designate diarrhea contracted during vacations in areas where hygiene is precarious: turista.

Travel morbidity[10] is mainly assessed by questionnaire surveys and by studies in travel medicine departments, with consultations before departure and on return. Due to the variety of methodologies and destinations, the proportion of travelers who fall ill varies from 15 to 70% across the different studies. In general, only 5 to 10% of travelers require medical attention during travel or upon return, but this figure may exceed 30% after return. More significantly, 5 in every 1,000 travelers are hospitalized (Caumes 2011). Traveler's diarrhea accounts for around half of all travel health problems, followed by ENT infections (ear infections, sinusitis, tonsillitis, colds), dermatitis (infectious and non-infectious), fever, accidents, motion sickness, altitude sickness and animal bites. These proportions vary according to the destination. For example, Bouchaud (2003) provides a table of the incidence of certain health events for a one-month stay in a developing country (Table 2.1).

Health event	Incidence
Any kind of health problem	60%
Traveler's diarrhea	40%
Bed rest	8%
Malaria (without chemoprophylaxis, in west Africa)	3%
Work stoppage on return	2%
Febrile respiratory infections	1.5%
Hospitalization abroad	0.4%
Hepatitis A	0.3%
Aeromedical evacuation	0.06%
Typhoid fever	0.003%
Death	0.001%
Cholera	0.0003%

Table 2.1. *Incidence of major health events among travelers (source: Bouchaud 2003)*

Turista, or traveler's diarrhea, is not an illness in itself. It is multifaceted and in medical terms it corresponds to different pathologies with the same symptom. It may or may not be infectious. It can be due to germs (the most common is *enterotoxigenic Escherichia coli*) or in around one case in five be of viral or

10 Morbidity refers to the state of illness or the frequency of illness.

parasitic origin. A simple change in eating habits can cause diarrhea in the first few days of a stay. Most often, the episode of turista occurs three to five days after arrival at the destination and disappears spontaneously within a few days, although there is a second peak in frequency around the 10th day. Turista is benign in the vast majority of cases.

Contamination occurs through the ingestion of contaminated food: fruits, raw vegetables, fish and seafood and drinking water. Personal hygiene is a determining factor, as well as the cleanliness of the accommodation: dirty hands and flies are significant vectors of pathogen agents. It is not always easy to control this hygiene, especially when eating in restaurants or from street stalls. There is no drug prophylaxis, so travelers are recommended to take some basic precautions to limit the risks: eat well-cooked meat, fish and shellfish (avoid rare steak and ground meat); avoid raw vegetables and fruits without husks and for the others, peel and wash them well before eating them; preferably drink water from sealed bottles or disinfect drinking water; wash your hands before each meal and when leaving the toilet; do not bathe just anywhere because the water is often contaminated with micro-organisms and do not forget that clear water is not necessarily biologically clean[11].

If, in spite of these precautions, the tourist falls ill, treatment is based primarily on good rehydration with a diet rich in sugar. Infectious diseases can be treated with intestinal antiseptics and antidiarrheal drugs.

Traveler's diarrhea is more of a nuisance than a serious problem for tourists in tropical countries. However, while the traveler usually gets off lightly and recovers quickly, the condition is more serious for local populations, especially children. Areas most at risk are in Southeast Asia, Africa and Latin America (Figure 2.8).

Africa and the Indian subcontinent are the two geographical areas most affected by the health risk related to poor access to drinking water, poor sanitation (wastewater, sewage, fecal matter treatment and so on) and hygiene (Figure 2.9). Figures vary widely between sources, but the WHO estimated in 2020 that these conditions related to poor water, sanitation and hygiene (WASH) are responsible for 2 million deaths per year, the majority of which are among children under the age of 5 years.

11 Recommendations from the Sante voyage guide: http://www.santevoyage-guide.com/zone-santevoyage/tourista.html, accessed 03/25/2020.

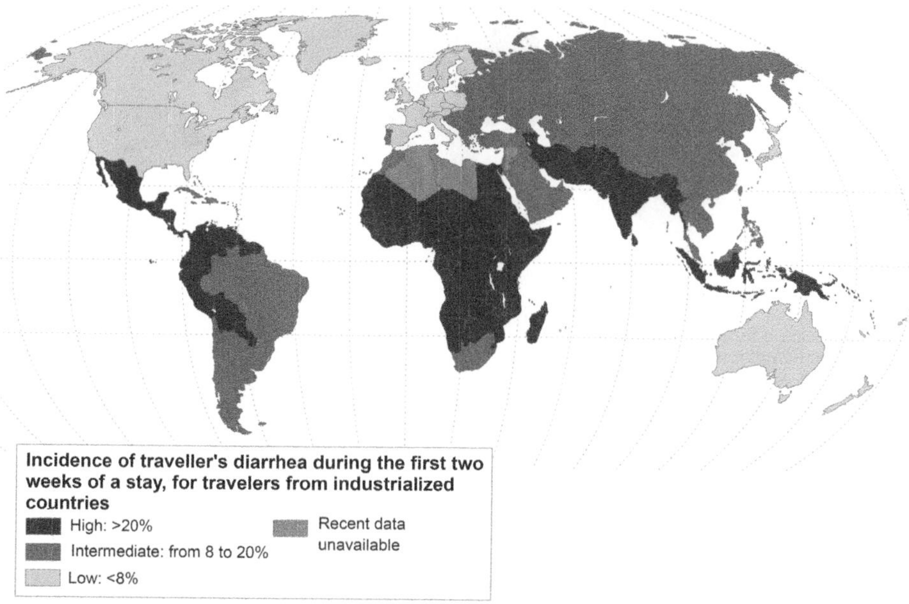

Figure 2.8. *Worldwide incidence of traveler's diarrhea (source: Steffen R., Hill D.R., Dupont H.L., Traveler's diarrhea: a clinical review, JAMA, 2015; background map: FNSP. Sciences Po – Cartography workshop CC BY 4.0; production: Lepetit A., UMR 6590 ESO)*

In addition to diarrhea, there are many diseases that are directly related to the issue of WASH, some of which are briefly listed below.

Cholera is a serious infectious disease caused by a bacterium (*Vibrio cholerae*). It is extremely virulent and can cause severe acute watery diarrhea that leads to rapid and fatal dehydration if not controlled. According to estimates (source: WHO), there are 1.3–4 million cases of cholera and 21,000–143,000 deaths each year. Contamination occurs through direct contact with the sick or by eating food that has been contaminated by their feces. This contamination from person to person causes episodic outbreaks.

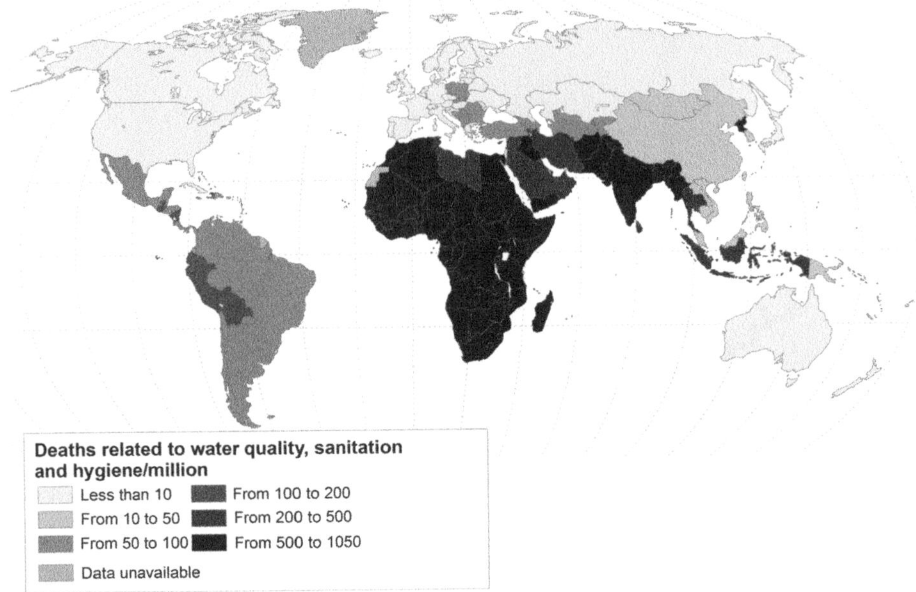

Figure 2.9. *Deaths due to poor access to water, hygiene and sanitation (source: World Health Organization, 2002. Map background: FNSP Sciences Po – Cartography workshop CC BY 4.0; production: Lepetit A., UMR 6590 ESO)*

The risk of contamination for travelers is extremely low and the best prevention is based on respecting hygiene rules. There is a vaccine, but it is not recommended for travelers except in the particular case of humanitarian tourism in high-risk places.

Typhoid and paratyphoid fever are typically orofecal transmission diseases related to poor hygiene. They are caused by bacteria belonging to the *Salmonella* genus, but whose reservoir is strictly human, and are very common in tropical environments, particularly Asia. According to the Institut Pasteur, contamination is most often the result of ingestion of water or food that has been contaminated by human feces or by direct person-to-person transmission. The symptoms are a high fever accompanied by headaches, abdominal pain and a feeling of despondency which gives the disease its name (*tuphos* in Greek means "torpor"). Treatment with antibiotics reduces mortality to less than 1% of cases, but instances of resistance to treatment have appeared in Southeast Asia and the Indian subcontinent. There are more than 20 million cases annually. There is a vaccination against typhoid fever that can be given to travelers: one injection protects for three years with a 60% protection rate in endemic areas (source: Institut Pasteur). Due to this limited protection rate, the vaccine does not replace the need to take precautionary measures regarding water and food[12].

Some viral hepatitis can be contracted by consuming contaminated food or water. These are hepatitis A and hepatitis E, two different diseases that affect the same organ: the liver. The risk of contamination is higher in tropical regions where these viruses are very present. There is a preventive vaccination for the hepatitis A virus, which is recommended for all travelers staying in a country with poor hygiene, whatever the conditions of the stay. People with chronic liver disease should be particularly protected by vaccination. There is no treatment for hepatitis E, which is self-limiting in most cases. However, as some forms of the disease can be severe, tourists traveling to high-risk areas should follow the basic rules of hygiene previously mentioned.

A final category of water, sanitation and hygiene-related diseases is digestive parasites. A number of parasitic diseases can be contracted by eating contaminated food. The main parasitic diseases are amebiasis and giardiasis and certain "intestinal worms".

Amebiasis is caused by the ameba *Entamoeba histolytica*, which is a parasite specific to humans. The particularity of this protozoan is that it forms cysts that proliferate in the intestine, some of which are expelled in stools and can thus contaminate other people if proper hygiene is not practiced. Amebiasis is most often asymptomatic but can, in some cases, cause painful and bloody diarrhea (amebic dysentery), ulcers and, in more severe forms, lead to abscesses in the liver, lungs and brain (source: Institut Pasteur). It is treated with broad-spectrum antiparasitics.

Giardiasis is an intestinal parasitosis caused by a single-cell parasite, *Giardia*. It is highly prevalent and present all over the world, including in industrialized countries, but is more common in hot and humid regions. Children are the most affected by this disease, which manifests itself through acute diarrhea, vomiting and abdominal pain. Treatment is based on the administration of an antiparasitic drug.

With regard to intestinal worms, there are far too many to be listed here without turning this book into a catalogue. Their treatment requires that they be properly identified, which makes it essential for the returning traveler seeking medical advice to list the countries visited and the fact that they were exposed to poor hygienic conditions in order to put their doctor on the trail and facilitate the diagnosis.

Tourists and tourism actors have a role to play in the fight against diseases related to water, sanitation and hygiene, by adopting prudent behaviors or by helping

12 Santé publique France, Weekly epidemiological bulletin no. 21-22 of 06/01/2010.

to promote good practices. This means everyday actions (e.g. to change behaviors), through the demand for higher hygiene standards by the tourism sector (which is spreading to other destinations) and, finally, through international programs such as UNICEF's WASH program.

In Madagascar, for example, around 8 million people, 37% of the population, still relieve themselves in the wild. Each year, half a million tons of excrement are expelled into the open air and constitute a significant source of contamination and disease linked to public insalubrity and to water pollution. Every year, tens of thousands of Malagasy, especially children under five, die from diarrhea, most of which is, in most cases, directly caused by impure water and lack of sanitation and hygiene. UNICEF Madagascar (through the WASH program), the tourism sector in five regions of the country, as well as actors in the water and sanitation sector, whether they are from the private or public sector or other structures, have therefore joined forces to launch a project to reduce this phenomenon. Hoteliers have been mobilized to communicate with communities about the need for latrines. The initiative was taken by hoteliers in the region of Tolagnaro (in the south of the island) and influenced other regions of Madagascar with the result that, according to UNICEF, 2,545,000 people have abandoned the practice of defecating in the wild.

In this Malagasy example, the tourism sector is doubly concerned: on the one hand, it benefits generally from the improvement in hygiene conditions, which promotes its development, and, on the other hand, it is participating in this improvement.

Another positive impact of tourism in the field of infectious diseases is that tourists who contract a disease can constitute a sentinel group and enable an epidemic to be measured in places where population monitoring cannot be carried out. The case of the schistosomiasis (otherwise known as bilharzia) in Dogon country provides a good example (Ranque et al. 2004).

The 1980s saw the development of tourist routes in Dogon country, in eastern central Mali. This geographical area is particularly isolated and the villages located at the foot of the Cliff of Bandiagara have neither water supply nor sanitation systems. The local populations use natural basins made of sandstone blocks at the foot of the cliff that fill with water during rainy periods, collecting runoff water from the plateau located at the top of the cliff. These natural basins are particularly attractive for tourists hiking in the Bandiagara Massif, and it is common for their guide to invite them to bathe there. This was the case for a group of Spanish travelers, reported by Ranque et al. (2004). The transmission of schistosomiasis during this swim was spectacular, as 28 of the 29 bathers in the tour group, who had only bathed once, were infested with one or more species of schistosomes. Schistosomiasis is a chronic parasitosis caused by worms (trematodes) of the genus *Schistosoma*, whose larvae penetrate a person's skin when in contact with infested water. If not treated properly, schistosomiasis can cause lesions in the urogenital system leading to sterility or liver and kidney damage. In children, it can cause anemia, which can lead to developmental delays.

The fact that tourists were affected in such a spectacular way put the spotlight on the problem of schistosomiasis in Dogon country. Epidemiological surveys were then conducted on the indigenous population, which revealed a prevalence of over 70% in the 7 to 14 age group. Mass treatments were then decided upon and, following this public health operation, lesions of the urinary tract decreased very significantly in this population. Thus, tourists acted as an indicator of the risk and the strength of the bilharzian infection (in epidemiology, this is known as a sentinel group). Travel medicine consultations following their infection also enabled clinical observations of primary infection, which is difficult to observe in the local population, who are often infected multiple times from early childhood, without necessarily consulting a doctor, given the scarcity of medical services in Dogon country.

Although in the above example the infection of tourists ultimately had a positive effect, the fact that, year after year, new cases of tourist groups contracting schistosomiasis are reported reflects a certain lack of tourist awareness of the health risks of traveling to tropical countries. Health recommendations appear to be too often focused on malaria and orofecal infections and neglect the risks related to parasitosis.

2.1.1.4. *Sexually transmitted infections (STIs)*

The link between tourism and sexually transmitted infections is, unlike other diseases, a widely studied subject (Halioua et al. 1997; Martet and Normand 2000; Tessier 2005), due, first, to its long history. In the past, sailors and soldiers were the main subjects of STIs: today, travelers are just ordinary people on vacation, the flesh is weak and the temptation to "do as they please" is present. Moreover, the subject of STIs is closely linked to the issue of sex tourism, which raises moral, ethical and legal questions, particularly when minors are the victims of practices that should be unequivocally condemned. UNICEF estimates that, each year, nearly 1 million children (mostly young girls) are forcibly recruited into the sex trade. The International Convention on the Rights of the Child, signed and ratified since 1989 by all countries except the United States, Somalia and South Sudan, stipulates in its article 34 that: "States Parties undertake to protect the child from all forms of sexual exploitation and sexual abuse." However, the prevention of STIs and reminders of the criminal nature of sex tourism involving minors are relatively absent from pre-travel medical consultations, where action is more focused on the return through screening, diagnosis and possible treatment. The French Federation of Tourism

Technicians and Scientists has published a guide to prevention and action against this scourge. It is available online: http://www.guide-fftst-ecpat.com.

Beyond the issue of protecting minors, sex tourism raises the question of the health of "sex workers" both mentally and emotionally, as well as physically (Garcia 2001). In a country like Thailand, the rate of HIV-AIDS infection among sex workers reached 70% in the 1990s.

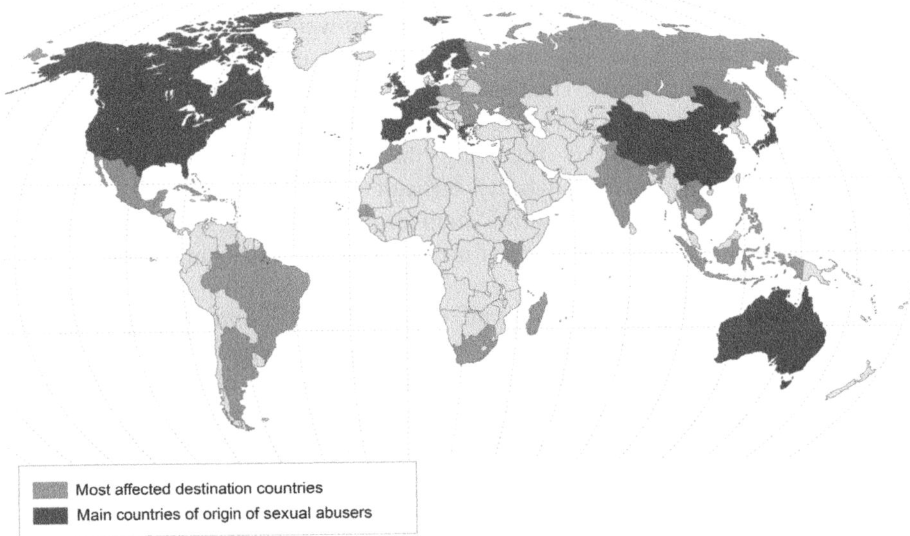

Figure 2.10. *Countries affected by sex tourism (source: ECPAT 2015; background map: FNSP. Sciences Po – Cartography workshop CC BY 4.0; production: Lepetit A., UMR 6590 ESO)*

The traveler is exposed to the risk of sexually transmitted infection, even when sex tourism is not involved. A study of a panel of young Australians (both male and female) vacationing alone to Thailand (Mulhall et al. 1993) found that a full one-third (34%) were considering having sex with a stranger during their stay, although sex was not the main reason for the trip.

When thinking of the risk of sexually transmitted infections, HIV/AIDS comes immediately to mind, but the list of STIs is long, as shown in the illustration below, which is taken from a health prevention document[13]. While it is possible to protect

13 This document is used by many health prevention and education organizations, but the original source is unknown to us.

against hepatitis B and human papillomavirus (HPV) infections[14] with a vaccine, the best protection against the rest of the "collection" (Figure 2.11) is condom use.

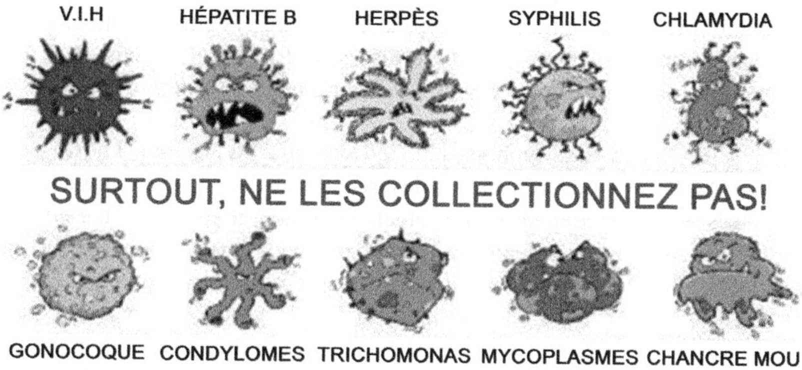

Figure 2.11. *Sexually Transmitted Infections prevention document, the text in red playing on tourist activity by stating "don't collect them!". From left to right the diseases are: HIV, hepatitis B, herpes, syphilis, chlamydia, gonorrhea, genital warts, trichomoniasis, mycoplasma and chancroid*

The human immunodeficiency virus (HIV) is responsible for acquired immunodeficiency syndrome (AIDS), which significantly weakens a person's immune system and makes them extremely vulnerable to many infections. An individual can be HIV positive without any symptoms of AIDS. Seropositivity is detectable three weeks after infection. The treatments for AIDS are complex and restrictive, even though significant progress has been made with the introduction of a triple therapy, which has greatly improved the vital prognosis of the infection. However, AIDS remains a serious disease and the risks of contamination during tourist stays remain high. A survey conducted in Quebec among travelers returning from a stay of less than two months (Tessier 2005) gives some orders of magnitude. In this study, one in ten tourists had sexual relations with a new partner during their trip, putting themselves at risk and only 69% of these people used a condom during sex. The majority had sex with a local person during their trip (55.6%), but 5.5% turned to prostitution, which is highly risky. Despite the fact that AIDS is a very well-known and documented disease, and that prevention messages are many and frequent, a significant proportion of the population is involved in risky behavior. Tourists can become infected and, on their return home, risk spreading the disease, as few of them are subsequently tested. International travel is an aggravating risk factor for

14 HPV causes genital warts (condyloma acuminata). These are highly contagious but harmless, except for certain varieties that lead to the appearance of precancerous lesions and then cervical cancer years later if no vaccine is given.

STIs. In addition, the growth and speed of air travel means that, today more than ever, travelers are more likely to return home during the incubation period of the infection they have contracted and are thus at risk of transmitting and spreading their STI in their country. In countries with a good healthcare system, and therefore a good system of detection and diagnosis of these diseases, it is estimated that 30% of new cases of syphilis are contracted overseas (De Schryver and Meheus 1989).

We have just mentioned syphilis and, indeed, other STIs, less known and less serious than AIDS, are nevertheless widespread, and the risk of contracting them during a tourist stay punctuated by unprotected sex is high. Some of these infections are viral, such as hepatitis B, genital herpes or condyloma (or genital warts) due to papillomavirus. Others are bacterial, such as syphilis, chlamydia, chancroid, gonococcus (or gonorrhea) and mycoplasma, while others are parasitic, such as trichomoniasis (vaginal infection). All these STIs weaken the mucous membranes and increase the risk of transmission of AIDS. They can all be treated, but those affected can be lifelong carriers of the herpes and hepatitis viruses without symptoms (and therefore put their partners at risk).

Some of these infections are also transmitted through blood, for example during a transfusion, and also during tattooing in uncontrolled sanitary conditions (see below) or through needle exchanges in the context of injecting drug use.

2.1.2. *Prevention is better than cure*

Travel medicine is both preventive and curative. However, its preventive aspect seems to need to be further developed as risky behaviors persist, and tourism professionals still seem to be largely unaware of the health issues that tourists may face.

In addition to pre-travel consultations, this prevention could be improved by a better knowledge of the geography of health risks on the model of what is already being done in terms of global security risk alerts. In France, for example, the Ministry of Foreign Affairs (MAE) publishes country-by-country recommendations in response to the political and health risks. It is possible to map the world according to health-related risks, as illustrated in the following map based on 2019 data (Figure 2.12, source: SOS International). The data used to categorize the different countries are: the significance of infectious diseases (and, if applicable, ongoing epidemics), a set of environmental factors, the standards and accessibility of emergency medical and dental services, the accessibility and quality of the pharmaceutical supply, the medical repatriation facilities, and any cultural, administrative or language barriers.

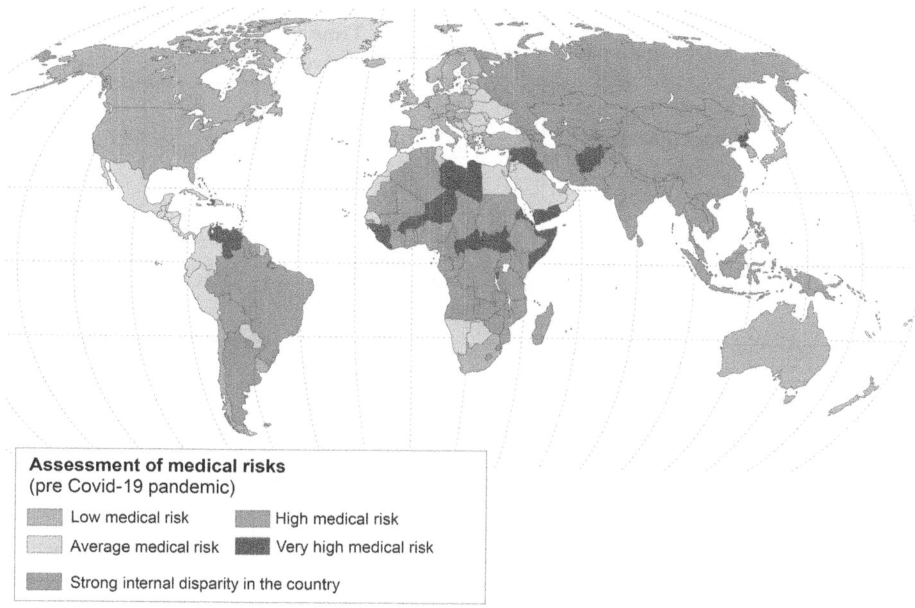

Figure 2.12. *The global health risk (source: SOS International, 2020; background map: FNSP. Sciences Po – Cartography workshop CC BY 4.0; design and production: Fleuret S., Lepetit A., UMR 6590 ESO)*

New technologies also offer opportunities for improving prevention and health while traveling. A study published in *Revue Médicale Suisse* (Genton and d'Acremont 2018) attempted a census of travel medicine smartphone apps and websites. Of the 29,000 Apple (IOS) and 21,000 Google (Android) apps classed as medical, three categories were identified:

– sites and apps for travel preparation, in the form of information (on the risks of infectious diseases, for example), recommendations or an electronic vaccination booklet;

– sites and apps providing travel advice, in the form of health guides, directories of health services, advice on food safety or real time information in case of a health crisis;

– post-travel care sites and apps, mainly for healthcare workers, which facilitate the diagnosis of "exotic" diseases for healthcare workers who rarely encounter these conditions and their symptoms.

Vaccine	Destinations	Mandatory	Time to travel	Validity	Minimum age
Yellow fever	Intertropical endemic area of Africa and Latin America	Yes	10 days	10 years	6 months
Meningitis	Meningitis belt (between 10 and 15 degrees north latitude in Africa)	Only for pilgrimages to Mecca	10 days	5 years	2 years
Japanese encephalitis	Southeast Asia, from Pakistan to the Philippines	No	10 days	2 years	1 year
Hepatitis A	Areas with poor hygiene	No	Immediate	10 years	1 year
Hepatitis B	High prevalence countries	No	1 month	10 years	None
Influenza	According to the seasons	No	A few days	Annual	6 months

Table 2.2. *Vaccines required before departure, by destination (source: INVS)*

One of the limitations of these types of tools is that, in order to be trusted, the information must be based on medical evidence, adequately referenced and regularly updated, which, according to the authors of the study, is not always the case; this calls the effective security of these applications into question. Other apps offer, for example, video consultations on a smartphone, which enables care to be accessed in medical deserts.

Finally, internet search engines today enable useful and practical information before a tourist stay to be found very quickly and easily. This is the case regarding information about vaccines, as illustrated in Table 1.2, which will certainly need to be updated and information added for the anti-Covid-19 vaccines, once the pandemic situation has stabilized.

2.2. Circulation of tourists, circulation of diseases

In a text entitled *Infectiologie itinérante*, Professor Rey (2007) judged, three years before the Covid-19 pandemic: "We must be aware of the current development of epidemics of severe infections. The considerable development of international transport has greatly amplified the circulation of infectious agents carried by travelers and migrants, but also by animals and goods. [...] This development requires a strengthening of international surveillance and alert response capabilities."

2.2.1. *International travel and the spread of epidemics*

The question of the circulation of diseases, punctuated by sometimes deadly epidemics, is part of a long history rich in research. Europe has, in the past, been hit several times by deadly epidemics, often imported by sea or land from the east (Rey 2007). Conversely, Europeans were able to spread certain diseases through their exploratory travel, colonization and later tourism. However, the spread of diseases through tourism is a poorly documented topic (Gössling 2005).

2.2.1.1. *The plague and cholera*

In the Middle Ages, it was the plague that was feared. In 1347, an epidemic of the Black Death, also known as the "Crimean Plague", swept through Europe. Its history reads like a novel. Not without anachronism, some evoke the first bacteriological warfare in history, combined with propagation through maritime navigation. The epidemic was indeed intentionally provoked by the Mongolian army that was besieging the Genoese colony of Caffa in Crimea. Struck down by the plague and forced to lift the siege, the Mongols catapulted their plague-ridden corpses over the walls of the city in order to exterminate the population within. Fleas and rats infested with the plague bacillus then embarked on Genoese ships bound for the west and spread the disease that would strike down nearly a third of the population of Europe. This epidemic led to the implementation of the first quarantine measures applied to ships. The plague landed in Italy and then embarked on all the commercial and maritime routes in order to contaminate the European territory, from coast to coast, from England to the Baltic Sea. This Crimean plague is therefore also considered the first historically documented global pandemic (Renouard 1948) and the first manifestation of the fact that diseases travel with humans.

Cholera, long known in Asia, arrived in Europe and America in the 19th century in successive epidemic waves. The bacillus responsible for the disease was only discovered in 1883 during the sixth of seven pandemic waves that punctuated history (Rey 2007). For a long time, the belief was that the disease was carried by miasmas in the air. Large fires of aromatic herbs were lit with a view to chasing them away, of course without success. During the 1848 epidemic in London, Dr John Snow had the idea of mapping the deaths and found that the concentration of cases in the Soho district decreased according to the distance from the Broad Street water pump; he had it closed and the epidemic died out in that neighborhood within a week. The door was opened to epidemiological studies and to the search for environmental causes of disease (in this case, orofecal transmission due to contamination of drinking water by seepage from the water from nearby latrines). As medicine progressed, it was understood that humans were vectors of this disease and that it was necessary, in addition to water sanitation, to interrupt the chains of contagion by isolating the vectors of propagation; soldiers, pilgrims, travelers and contaminated migrants. Thus, in 1887, the first systematic screening of new arrivals in New York (United States) was implemented.

Cholera is an opportunity to address a particular type of tourism: religious tourism and, more particularly, pilgrimage. Indeed, pilgrimages to Mecca have been proven to contribute to the international dissemination of this disease. Imported by Indian and Javanese Muslims, the disease spread rapidly among the dense crowds of pilgrims, causing the deaths of more than a third of them in 1865. Thereafter, cholera spread worldwide as pilgrims returned to their countries of origin. Steam navigation and the railroad, modern and fast means of transportation, had introduced a novelty: people now traveled faster than the incubation periods and the weather, which played the role of a prophylactic barrier by slowing down the dissemination (Chantre 2013), had lost this function. Even today, major pilgrimages are monitored for health concerns and the meningitis vaccination is required, for example, when traveling to Mecca during the annual grand pilgrimage. More recently, a cholera epidemic broke out in Yemen in the midst of the civil war (in 2017) and caused the WHO to fear that it would spread to Mecca, justifying the issuance of an official alert. In their alert, the WHO noted that pilgrimage brings together several million people in a small space, half of whom are foreigners, thus providing an ideal setting for the spread of diseases such as meningitis, yellow fever, dengue or zika, as well as cholera.

2.2.1.2. *From Spanish flu to avian flu*

Influenza is well known as a seasonal epidemic, but it also occasionally strikes in the form of pandemics whose spread follows international travelers. The best known was Spanish flu[15] (H1N1) which, at the end of World War I, spread worldwide due to the movement of military troops. It is estimated to have caused between 20 and 40 million deaths, more than the war itself. Other influenza epidemics have punctuated the history of the 20th century: Asian flu (H2N2) in 1957, Hong Kong flu (H3N2) in 1968 and, more recently, another flu has put the world on pandemic alert: avian flu (H5N1). Once identified and spread in the population, influenza viruses only cause seasonal epidemics, and an annual vaccination prevents their severity in the most fragile people. Nevertheless, new viral strains emerge at regular intervals and the population has no immunity because human organisms have never been

15 Spanish flu actually originated in the United States, but it got its name because Spain was the only country to publish public health data (other countries, then involved in World War I, hid this data).

confronted with them and have not had the opportunity to produce antibodies. The SARS-CoV-2 coronavirus that caused the Covid-19 pandemic in 2020 (see above) is a perfect illustration. However, to fully understand the impact of this crisis, we must remember previous episodes and, in particular, the fears caused by avian flu, which was due to the H5N1 virus that infects birds and has been circulating since 2003 in many Asian countries. In some cases, it can be transmitted to humans (in poultry farms or by eating undercooked infected meat), although human-to-human transmission of H5N1 is low. Between November 2003 and December 2009, however, 467 human cases of avian flu were reported in 15 countries (WHO) with a high mortality rate (285 deaths). The fear that the virus would mutate to adapt to humans was strong, leading to drastic preventive measures such as the slaughter of entire poultry farms upon discovery of the slightest suspect case in the vicinity. The brutality of these measures in the face of the low number of cases left its mark on public opinion, especially since, in 2009, a new H1N1-type of influenza appeared, whose virus was a combination of avian, swine and human influenza. The virus would have emerged in a pig farm in Mexico or Asia (experts do not agree on this point) and would then have spread across the world, propagated by international travelers (125 countries would be affected). In response to the spread of this virus, and out of fear of a major pandemic causing several million deaths (a number of WHO officials were particularly alarmist at the time), many countries (including Australia, China, India, Indonesia, Malaysia, the Philippines, Singapore, Thailand, South Korea and Iceland) instituted surveillance of travelers coming from affected areas, which involved temperature checks (detection of fevers) and testing for symptoms of respiratory disorders. Many other countries have put in place measures to inform travelers and encourage them to seek medical attention immediately in case of flu-like symptoms. Other countries have banned the import and sale of pork. Finally, estimates of the number of deaths related to this flu vary from 18,000 to 200,000, this lack of accuracy being due to the fact that many cases are confused with seasonal flu. However, the most important thing to consider going forward is not the number of deaths, but rather the treatment of the crisis. Following the announcement of the pandemic (the European Union would later reproach the WHO for having exaggerated the extent of the crisis), many countries set up vaccination plans using very different strategies. France chose to seek to reach a collective immunity threshold of around 75% of the population vaccinated. It was not the only country to make this choice: Canada, for example, made the same decision. However, the implementation of these mass vaccination plans was rushed and there were many problems. In addition, vaccines are relatively expensive, and, because of the massive nature of the orders (all affected countries were simultaneously submitting the same demands), some of the doses would arrive late, once the epidemic was over. Anti-vaccine groups needed no second invitation to pounce: complaints were filed against the health authorities for collective poisoning, and rumors circulated, relayed by the media, which were a priori very serious. The newspaper *Le Monde* published a British study accusing the anti-flu drug “Tamiflu” of causing nausea and nightmares in children. Rumors, amalgams and mockery flourished, and the Minister of Health was accused of having preventively overreacted to a "mini flu" by the same people who would accuse her successors of not having done enough in the face of Covid-19.

This episode in the world history of diseases is crucial because in some countries health authorities would be discredited and distrust instilled in public opinion as regards health warnings; and just like in the children's story in which, after having cried wolf several times for fun, little Peter is not believed the day he is really attacked, many countries, including France, would approach the Covid-19 pandemic insufficiently prepared and have a hard time accepting the lockdown measures decided upon to stop the contagion.

The global epidemics have highlighted a number of major issues. The first is the control of the circulation of viruses, which is extremely complex in a world where goods and tourists move in all directions, over great distances and over extremely short timescales. In addition to this, there is the circulation of information, and also (and especially) misinformation ("fake news"), which is also extremely rapid and favored by the Internet and by the interculturality which has facilitated the globalization of international exchanges. It should be an asset in the effective dissemination of warning and prevention messages: unfortunately, it seems to be a handicap and is diminishing the acceptance of health instructions by a significant part of the population, convinced that they are dealing with a global conspiracy hatched by the pharmaceutical industry (which is not exempt from any reproach, but that is another story).

"Travel, as a factor in the spread of disease, falls within the domain of public health research" (Rodriguez-Garcia 2001) However, the tourism industry has been short-sighted in this area and has completely failed to integrate health risks into its development models, including the risk relating to the need to stop the international flow of people in order to contain the spread of disease. SARS and then Covid-19 have brought this to light, and it appears that, today a globalized reflection must be carried out in order to isolate, trace and contain developing cases and block their spread, which resolutely inscribes health in international transport and especially tourism policies. At present, visas and authorizations to enter territories are issued on economic and political grounds; in the future, health criteria may be added.

2.2.2. *Non-infectious risks and diseases: travel-related variations*

"The rapid growth of tourism has led to an increased need for health training and education tailored to ensure safe and healthy travel. While advice in this area typically focuses on behaviors to address preventable [that is to say, infectious] diseases, it rarely includes the environmental health risks to which tourists may be exposed." (Bauer 2001) According to Bauer, tourism studies typically point to the (often negative) impacts of tourism on the environment, but not the impacts of the environment on the health of tourists, because, she argues, tourists and the environment are treated as two separate entities when, in fact, they interact. It is therefore necessary to change the way in which we look at things.

2.2.2.1. *Understanding and knowledge of environmental risk*

Apart from the water-related risks already mentioned, which are a link between environmental and infection risks, it is possible to identify and list several categories of environmental risk to which tourists may be exposed during their stay, without necessarily being located in a particularly hostile area.

The diversity of exposure factors and the assessment of associated risks require

> a huge epidemiological effort that has yet to be undertaken. These studies are difficult to carry out due to the significant number of travelers to be included, which is necessary to identify and evaluate risks whose probability of occurrence remains low. [...] Given the enormous costs, these types of studies are now very difficult to carry out [...]. Moreover, these studies are essentially interested in a "general" population, whereas they should focus on more specific categories of travelers, taking into account the type of travel (sports trips, isolation situations and so on), and particularities of the "field" (such as elderly people, diabetics, pregnant women and children). For the same reasons of cost, studies evaluating preventive strategies are also difficult to carry out (Bouchaud 2003).

Despite these difficulties in quantifying the phenomenon and applying it to travel medicine, it is possible to identify risk factors associated with tourism.

First, tourist travel is often synonymous with a change of environment, which means loss of reference points, habits and reflexes. It can also confront the tourist with unknown risks since, as Cossar (1995) points out, travel exposes the individual to new cultural, psychological, physiological, physical, emotional, environmental and microbiological experiences.

It starts on the journey. Motion sickness is the mildest form and is usually reflected in simple dizziness and nausea, which can, however, make a journey particularly unpleasant. It is caused by a mismatch between two pieces of information sent to the brain: one from the eyes, the other from the inner ear. When either indicates movement (the landscape while moving) and the other perceives stillness (sitting on a boat, plane, train or car), then symptoms emerge. The discomfort is all the more pronounced when the transport is more agitated: for instance, seasickness increases with the swell. The body usually becomes used to motion sickness, which disappears in a few minutes at the end of the journey. There are some recommended remedies: airing the cabin whenever possible, looking at a fixed point on the horizon to resynchronize the eyes and the inner ear and so on. Prophylactic medicines are available, but, due to the risk of inappropriate use, travelers must consult a doctor rather than resort to self-medication.

There are more serious risks related to transport and particularly to air transport. To fly at a cruising altitude above 10,000 meters, cabins need to be pressurized, changing the atmospheric pressure inside the aircraft. This does not pose any problem for healthy individuals, but creates risks due to a too low oxygen supply[16] for people suffering from respiratory insufficiency, severe anemia or for pregnant women, for example. Respiratory assistance may then prove necessary and a hypoxic test before the trip will enable this need to be determined.

Another serious risk is that of thrombosis (phlebitis), the formation of a blood clot in the venous network, which, in its most serious forms, can cause a potentially fatal pulmonary embolism. Its frequency during air travel is low (less than 100 cases per million travelers[17]), but the risk increases with the duration of the flight: from zero risk below 4 hours, it becomes significant above 8 hours, particularly for subjects at risk, for example, people with a history of venous disease such as arterial hypertension (who are often well informed of this risk by their doctors), obese people, pregnant women, heavy smokers and diabetics[18]. Contrary to popular belief, the risk is as high in business class as in economy class since it is principally related to immobility. On the contrary, an aisle seat is less risky than a window seat, because it is easier to get up and move around the plane. Dehydration due to dry air in pressurized cabins and the decrease in oxygen levels in the atmosphere are the two other risk factors. Some cases of phlebitis occur up to 14 days after the return journey, but can still be attributed to the journey. It is therefore advisable for everyone, and not only those at risk for flights longer than 8 hours, to take a few precautions: to wear compression stockings, since thrombosis mainly affects the lower limbs, to move around regularly on board, in order to take breaks from immobility, and to stay well hydrated.

16 The conditions during air travel are similar to those encountered at an altitude of 1,500–2,500 meters, which represent decreases in oxygen partial pressure and oxygen blood saturation.

17 Nevertheless, we should recall the distrust of the anti-Covid Astra Zeneca vaccine for a risk 20 times lower!

18 This list is not exhaustive.

Changes in atmospheric pressure can also affect tourists during certain sporting activities that we will discuss later (mountaineering or scuba diving).

Air travel and speed over long distances are also responsible for a discomfort that can impact the health of travelers in varying degrees, without having serious consequences: jet lag is a disruption of the internal clock that usually controls the body's circadian rhythms (24-hour cycles). It occurs following rapid travel through several time zones and can, in addition to fatigue, cause physical symptoms, such as digestive disorders, constipation, daytime sleepiness and reduced physical and mental performance. These symptoms fade over time, as the body adapts to its new rhythm, and are not serious. Nevertheless, they can cause alertness deficits that become risky for certain activities (extreme sports, for example). There is no way to prevent jet lag, but it is possible to reduce its effects, such as by adapting rhythms before the trip or by adjusting diet. However, the WHO warns people with chronic illnesses, or who are on daily medication or contraceptives, to be vigilant when adjusting the rate of their medication intake. A prior consultation with a travel medicine specialist may be appropriate.

Once at the destination, the tourist faces other changes in their environment. Extreme temperature variations can cause hypo- or hyperthermia following prolonged outdoor activities. The press regularly reports cases of varying degrees of severity of hypothermia[19] in tourists who have gone mountain hiking without appropriate clothing and who find themselves exposed to the sudden changes in weather that are common in these environments (such as fog, storms or snow). Swimming also exposes them to the risk of hypothermia. Conversely, heat waves and certain particularly arid and hot areas (such as Death Valley in California) expose tourists to the risk of hyperthermia[20], which occurs when the body can no longer regulate body temperature, causing headaches, dizziness, nausea and even heart failure. Children and the elderly are particularly at risk. Also, certain sports activities (running or cycling in hot weather, hiking in desert or arid areas, swimming during the hottest hours of the day) can expose the risk of hyperthermia and cause dehydration in the body, which will be aggravated in case of travel diarrhea or excessive alcohol consumption.

In these examples, we can see that the main factors for preventing health risks are ultimately consultation of weather reports and adaptation of the intensity of activities, as well as foresight (to take equipment, food and adapted clothing on excursions, for example).

---

19 Reduction in body temperature, which can lead to loss of consciousness and death.

20 The risk from the sun is discussed further in a section on body standards, which notably includes tanning in beach tourism.

Adaptation to environmental conditions during a tourist stay and, by extension, attitudes and behaviors, can be risk factors. Literature points to a relaxation of attention during vacations which can lead a person to place themself in risky situations that they would not have experienced in normal daily life. According to Cossar (1995), for example, the relaxed attitudes and reduction of inhibitions that are a natural part of the pleasure of vacations expose the traveler to risk. Bauer (2001) writes that even though the responsibility should not be all placed on the individual, the sick tourist is not always an innocent victim. In many cases, it is the culpable behavior of tourists that has put their health at risk. Thus, when we talk about an incident caused by environmental factors, we must distinguish between what is ignorance, risk taking and what is a real and unforeseeable accident. Page and Meyer (1996) refer to the importance of employee training in first aid and safety, the management of accident prevention systems, pre-established procedures and legislative provisions which, depending on their adequacy, can affect the probability of accidents occurring, and also their consequences and severity.

Among the high-risk activities are sports activities. Vacations are often an opportunity to indulge in activities that are a little out of the ordinary, without preparing for them by physical training, for example. Many winter sports accidents occur at the end of the stay, when tired muscles are less performant and less resistant. At the seaside, scuba diving can also be cited as an example of an activity with quite significant risks, such as the less serious skin lacerations (on sharp rocks, for example) and stings (from sea urchins, for example), or the more serious decompression accidents and drowning (Bauer 2001). Even minor injuries can have unfortunate consequences that the poorly informed tourist discovers at their expense. Marine injuries can easily be infected by bacteria in sea water, and no major trauma is required to cause a serious infection.

While also alerting us to the accident risk factors linked to a poor understanding of the environment, Page and Meyer (1996) nevertheless qualify the importance of the risk by pointing out that barely more than 1% of international tourists are victims of an accident reported during their stay.

Moreover, while certain activities practiced during tourist stays can cause accidents, they can also indirectly, through this risk, be the reason for the establishment of health services. One example is a first-aid post set up on a scuba diving site, with a nurse and basic equipment that will also be used to treat the local population in a place previously devoid of any health services. In some tourist destinations, such as winter sports resorts, medical facilities (such as an X-ray room) have been set up where the population density would normally be too low to justify such a facility, but which is therefore entirely the result of the influx of tourists and sports activities with a high trauma risk. In the same way, emergency health services and evacuation facilities (such as ambulances and helicopters) can be set up in a destination because of its tourist appeal and to benefit the population. In France, the coastline of the Provence-Alpes-Côte-d'Azur region is one of the best-endowed regions in the country in terms of medical density, due to the combined presence of summer tourists and numerous senior citizens, who come to spend all or part of their retirement in the sun and who constitute an attractive patient base for health professionals (even though, as we will see later, tourism is not sufficiently taken into account in regional health planning schemes – see Chapter 5).

Finally, another risk factor linking the understanding of the environment and health results in a lack of knowledge of the biophysical environment. The resulting risks are classified as biological risks. These may be animal bites or stings from local fauna of which tourists may be unfamiliar and have not learned to be wary, in some cases the consequences can be serious. Rabies is the main risk in terms of diseases but fortunately a vaccine exists. In relation to the context, it is not the same animals that carry the highest risk. The urban tourist will be wary of stray dogs, whereas in the Amazon, 100% of rabies cases among tourists in the forest are due to bats (Bauer 2001). Some animals are venomous (snakes, spiders, scorpions and so on): in Australia, for example, nearly 3,000 snake bites are reported each year. Depending on the species, some bites are more toxic than others, and the resulting risk of fatality varies. Generally speaking, the problem is greater in the most remote areas where the tourist does not have rapid access to medical services, for example, during mountain hikes or excursions in the desert. However, misfortune can also occur in the context of coastal tourism, where there is no extreme characteristic. For example, more than 500,000 jellyfish stings are reported each year at Chesapeake Bay in the United States, which cause localized reactions (hives, inflammation, blisters, itching, necrosis) and, in some cases, more serious reactions, such as anaphylactic shock or toxicity to organs such as the heart, kidneys or respiratory system, depending on the level of toxicity of the sting (Bauer 2001).

The biological risk can also be vegetal and results in irritations, or even cases of poisoning by unknown plants. It is not uncommon for French tourists visiting Quebec to come into contact with plants while walking in the forest, without knowing (since they do not exist in their own country) that there are two varieties known respectively as poison ivy (*Toxicodendron radicans*), which is responsible for dermatitis when touched, and ragweed (*Ambrosia artemisiifolia*), the pollen of which causes rhinitis-like respiratory reactions, similar to hay fever (Figure 2.13).

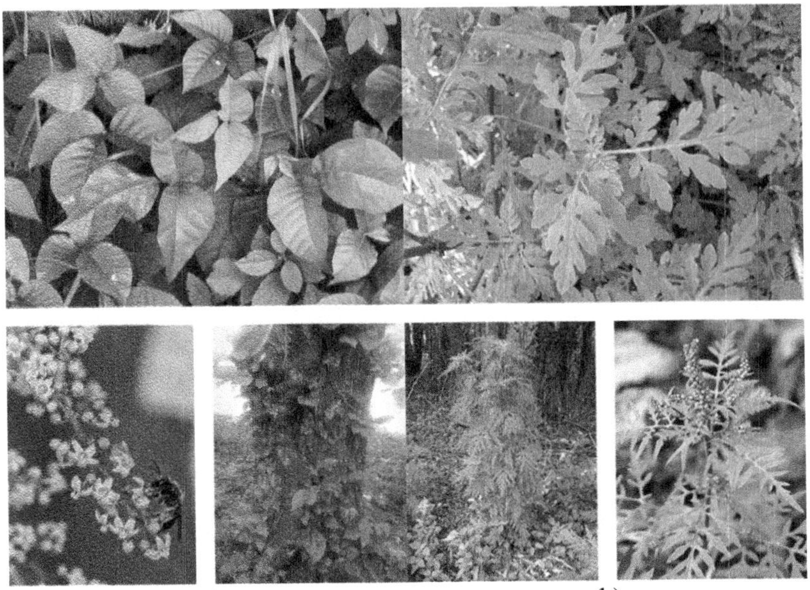

a) b)

Figure 2.13. *a) Ragweed and b) poison ivy (source: sciencepresse.qc.ca)*

Traveling therefore exposes us to contact with unusual species, from which the body is not protected by progressive immunization and which we are not aware of during certain seemingly harmless activities, such as country picnics or the picking of wild flowers.

The lessons of the lack of understanding and knowledge of environmental risks for health observed among tourists are posed in terms of communication. In tourist areas, it is necessary to carry out a survey of the dangers and to develop prevention and health education (action on individual behavior) documents and to involve the tourist industry in the prevention of and response to possible accidents. These communication issues must clearly be dissociated from the temptation to minimize the danger, particularly when the environmental risk is concomitant with an epidemiological risk, and when there is a great fear of "scaring away tourists", and thus harming economic activity (Gössling 2005).

2.2.2.2. *Travel and mental health*

Like all health social sciences, mental health is a field that is, to say the least, under-investigated. Yet, "travel is a stress that can reveal or aggravate a mood disorder, a specific anxiety disorder or a substance abuse problem" (Eytan and Loutan 2006). "Faced with novelty, a progressive reorganization in our relationship with ourselves and the world takes place" (Dutray and Moulins 2005). Mental health problems during travel range from minor problems of adaptation to a new context to acute psychotic episodes and anxiety attacks. In relation to the number of international tourists, the prevalence of psychotic disorders among travelers is limited, but it still represents 10–20% of the reasons for health repatriation (Vermersch et al. 2014). Certain destinations are particularly associated with a greater frequency of more or less acute psychotic episodes due to their symbolic or mystical connotations.

In this area, it is important to distinguish different situations: psychiatric disorders may occur during or after a trip in people who had no previous problems; patients who are being treated for psychiatric disorders may go on a trip, their pathology having stabilized; some may "decompensate" during their trip (Airault 2011). Moreover, variations can be observed according to the nature and the duration of the trip in question (many studies include migrants and expatriates). We will limit ourselves here to discussing travel for tourism purposes, which can sometimes resemble therapeutic travel: the tourist expects a change of scene, by going to a sunny destination, for example, in order to escape winter seasonal depression, to improve the disorders from which they are suffering. At the end of the 19th century, it was common to treat melancholy in this way, and in North America, the name "snowbirds" is given to the inhabitants of the north of the continent who go to the tropics (such as Florida, Cuba or Santo Domingo) to escape the rigors of winter.

A first category of mental health disorders related to travel results from the loss of reference points and the phase shift that strikes the subject who is plunged into a world in which they find nothing familiar. This can occur in a wide variety of situations: confrontation with extreme poverty, the observation of rites or customs that provoke a culture shock, or simply a situation of distancing from the usual supports (such as loved ones or parents) that destabilize the tourist. These disorders are often minor, but can generate anxiety, depression, somatic symptoms and, in the most serious cases, suicidal behaviors (Stewart and Leggat 1998).

A second category includes mood disorders and psychoses which may have several causes, including fatigue, particularly that linked to jet lag, as mentioned above, some symptoms of which occasionally resemble a depressive episode. Another cause may be the occurrence of anxiety attacks (these are usually the first to emerge, since people with chronic anxiety disorders tend to avoid traveling). Fear of flying can also initiate mood disorders or even psychoses. Finally, there are reports of manic episodes (states of overexcitement or even exaltation) in people with bipolar disorders, which are exacerbated by the fatigue associated with travel.

In addition, people on psychotropic drugs whose treatment has not been re-evaluated prior to the trip may find that their situation worsens. Finally, some prophylactic treatments, such as mefloquine (malaria prevention), have adverse side effects, such as anxiety, depression or hallucinations, most often in people with a psychiatric history (Eytan and Loutan 2006).

Finally, the controversial issue of pathological travel and destinations that may lead to psychiatric hospitalizations must be addressed. In many cases, these are patients whose "delusions of mystical, persecutory or vindictive themes are responsible for psychiatric disorders in these patients" (Eytan and Loutan 2006). Thus, several syndromes, often related to the destination, have been described. They are sometimes grouped under the term "traveler syndromes"[21]. Certain destinations seem to be more conducive than others to the onset of psychotic symptoms in travelers, particularly those with particular meanings that the traveler has "fantasized" about before their stay. During the trip, an individual may have a destabilizing experience if, by chance, there is too great a distinction between imagination and reality.

For example, it is estimated that about 100 travelers each year suffer from "Jerusalem syndrome", an acute psychotic state with a religious theme (Bar-el et al. 2000). Sightseeing is said to be the triggering event for this syndrome, which occurs without any substance use or major stress. People affected by this syndrome feel the need to go to holy places and to chant, haranguing the crowd in a speech that resembles a confused sermon.

Another example is that psychopathological manifestations have been observed among tourists during a visit to the city of Florence in Italy, which are referred to as the "Stendhal syndrome" in reference to an episode experienced by the author Stendhal in Florence when leaving the Santa Croce church. It is a state of intense ecstasy accompanied by a strong emotional charge when in the presence of a work of art.

"Paris syndrome" is similar, but seems to operate principally among Japanese tourists. Paris and Florence are the only two cities in Europe that offer specialized assistance in Japanese to these travelers who present delusional syndromes with mystical, erotomanic or persecutory themes (Ota 1988).

"Geneva syndrome" affects travelers with persecutory delusions who may travel to the Swiss city to contact international organizations such as the UN or the WHO.

---

21 The clinical picture of these syndromes is described in the article by Vermersch *et al.* (2014), referenced in the bibliography. We do not detail it here.

"Ulysses syndrome" may be observed among long-distance travelers who leave for several months[22], which occurs following the return from a trip. Individuals experience difficulties in readapting to their environment and their culture of origin and feel like strangers in places that were once familiar to them. This can lead to a period of depression and requires a mourning process of grieving for the journey in order to "find a place that no longer exists at home" (Airault 2011). For many, the temptation to leave is great.

Finally, there are various syndromes linked to places of pilgrimage such as Mecca, Santiago de Compostela or certain sacred places in India, which is moreover the subject of a study that focuses more on minor mental disorders than on acute episodes (Dutray and Moulins 2005). For its authors, "the emotional pathway during a trip to India would be the intersection of the myths of *terra incognita* and the experience of disturbing strangeness. [...] In order to complete the 'imagined journey', each person adopts and also conforms to 'postures', which represent a desire to fit in with an imaginary and an ideal of the journey". However, as the study describes, the traveler finds themselves confronted with the reality and the frustrations of travel: sometimes lost in the crowd, sometimes isolated confused by the behavior of the Indians, which is at the same time familiar and so different. These travelers who had imagined themselves arriving in a country full of harmony and spirituality are confronted with a certain disillusionment that sometimes borders on rejection accompanied by stress and somatic disorders. The oppressive crowd, the contacts and promiscuity, the poverty and pollution are, according to Dutray and Moulins, felt as aggressions and the positive vision of the journey is reversed, provoking a feeling of anger and even sometimes hatred.

The psychiatrist R. Airault (2000) maintains that "India can drive westerners crazy", and, in these situations, "most of the time a return to the country of origin is necessary in order to regain a foothold on the reality to which the subject was initially shaped".

To conclude on this point, it is important to consider the potential aggravating factors of alcohol, drugs and other psychotropic substances. It is not uncommon for certain mystical travel experiences to be accompanied by the consumption of these products, sometimes under the "supervision" or influence of neoshamanism, with the abuses that this can entail, to which we will return later in this work.

---

22 An entire passage in this book is dedicated to backpackers and "round-the-worlders" (section 3.4).

2.2.3. *Travel mortality and its causes*

The risk of death while traveling is estimated at 1 in 100,000 (Caumes 2011). The main causes of death during tourist stays are accidental and traumatic (especially traffic accidents), for almost half, or, in more than a quarter of cases, cardiovascular in nature (Dioko and Harrill 2019). Infectious diseases account for just over one in a hundred deaths, and the only tropical disease with any notable visibility in these statistics is malaria resulting from non-compliance with prophylactic treatments.

The topic of death is little studied in the field of tourism, outside of researching causes of death in travel medicine, and another topic: macabre tourism, also known as dark tourism. Pratt et al. (2019) have, in fact, called for more research in this area in an article published in the journal *Annals of Tourism Research*. Indeed, while death is not supposed to be part of the tourism experience and while we prefer "not to think about it" because the tourism stay is, above all, a positive experience, a better knowledge of mortality factors, even though it concerns a small number of people, could contribute to an improvement in the prevention of risks during travel. Improving the management of the repatriation of a body, the accompanying announcement of the death and the mourning process are also areas to be explored.

Finally, the apprehension of death, the resulting fear, its nature and its extent, which may vary according to destination and culture, are also likely to provide information on the behavior of tourists and, in particular, their propensity to take risks or not, depending on their perception of the danger.

2.2.4. *Health upon return home (example of post-travel depression)*

Post-return depression is one of the manifestations, which varies depending on the individual, of the identity adjustment that occurs during any life transition, such as a return from a trip. Some people are not subject to it at all (about 30–40% of the population, according to the groups studied), while some (between 60 and 70% of the population) experience it as a slight and temporary depression, while others, depending on their personal, family and social trajectory, may experience a real depression that is all the more pronounced depending on the length of their trip.

Fortunately, not everyone who comes back from a trip is subject to depression[23]. For some, there may be a "slump" linked to a brutal transition between two environments and two rhythms of life, all of which may be amplified by fatigue and

23 Be aware, depression is an illness. It is different from the "blues", or a simple bout of feeling low. It must be treated by a health professional without delay and be the subject of a professional diagnosis (not self-diagnosis).

stress. Depression describes a depressive state that lasts several weeks or months, during which the person closes themselves off from the outside world in a state of suffering that nothing really relieves.

Post-return depression is often experienced in people who return from a world tour or a tourist trip lasting several months, especially if this return was not prepared for by anticipating a return to a sedentary lifestyle, a work rhythm and so on. There is care suited to this problem and even, for example, in France, a guide for returning expatriates which can be useful for long-term tourists.

2.3. Bodies, tourism activities and health

> The body constitutes the first level of the spatiality of individuals. [...] It is the place by and through which each individual enters into relation with the world that surrounds him, the skin constituting an interface between interiority and exteriority, a 'spatial object' enabling each person to experience the limit between the inner and the outer, the subjective and the objective. (Coëffé et al. 2019)

The body is at the forefront of tourism activities. Throughout history, it has, first, been a case of caring for it, by bathing it, applying hygiene to it, then maintaining it through physical activities, even shaping it, and finally by relaxing and unwinding it, through rest and massages or simply by warming it up in the sun on a beach. Our relationship with the body has evolved over time: from dressed baths to naturism, from conserving a milky complexion to tanning, until we are now, in certain cases, at a veritable worship of the body highlighted by prominent musculature or tattoos, for example.

2.3.1. *The relationship with the sun and how new body norms emerge*

For a long time, tanning was, in western societies, seen as a negative marker of bodies, the stigma of low-wage outdoor work. Ory (2008) speaks of an "ancient epidermal regime", during which the peasant displayed a tanned complexion, while the aristocrat opted to have skin as white as possible to indicate his belonging to the higher social classes of those who did not have to submit to lowly tasks. The good and the beautiful were pale and smooth, the bad and the ugly were dull or leathered. The advent of tourism, and more specifically coastal tourism, changed this over the course of history. The slogan "sea, sand and sun" has established a tourism model that is different from the original practices of care and rest, leading to the emergence of new destinations and causing some other, too northern, destinations to pass out of fashion. As the MIT researchers write (2011), "over the long term, the tourist's body fundamentally changes through a long process that will operate a shift in dominant values: from white to tanned, from hidden to naked, from established practices to advanced practices [...]. The history of tourism related to the body has been one of the advents of pleasure leading to self-esteem throughout the body". Very recently, the question of health has resurfaced in this history of tourism related to the body in several ways: through the discovery of the risks linked to the sun, through the idealization of a model of a healthy body (we might ask ourselves whether this model is really new or ancient) or through the generalization of certain practices that were previously confined to minority groups, such as tattooing.

This return to the issue of health does not mean placing resting of the body in the hands of doctors during the tourist experience, but, rather, as part of a global vision of health and its determinants, to consider how it influences practices.

Let us take a moment to consider how our relationship with the sun has helped shape body norms over the past two centuries.

The 19th century saw the emergence of a trend in naturist alternative medicine which developed primarily in Germany and Austria, in Gräfenberg, for example, where a center of hydrotherapy advocated care by the exposure of naked skin to cold water. Later that century, the emergence of heliotherapy, advocated in the treatment of tuberculosis, among other things, resulted in the recommendation of sunbathing in sanatoriums (as previously discussed), which replaced hydrotherapy. Through this heliotherapy, which has now fallen into disuse, the hygienist school of thought emphasized the benefits of exposing the body to light, which was based both on scientific principles and on a certain therapeutic idealization. Although the scientific beliefs on which heliotherapy was based have since been proven wrong, the reality of the physiological effects of exposure to sunlight is now proven: the production of vitamin D, for example, results from exposure to ultraviolet (UV) rays. In summer and spring, 10–20 minutes of exposure to the sun each day enables sufficient production of vitamin D, but in winter, the time required to synthesize the same quantity is around 2 hours, because UV radiation is weaker and because, on average, only 10% of the body is uncovered during the winter season, which limits exposure. The positive influence of the sun on blood circulation and the immune system also form part of the arguments in favor of sunbathing advocated by heliotherapy. However, it is all a matter of exposure time, as the sun can become "our health's own worst enemy" (Andrieu 2011), as we will see later. Heliotherapy was also based on the therapeutic idea of storing solar energy in the body. The skin was then seen as "a field of exchange between the body and the natural environment" (Bauberot 2008). This vision met with a certain degree of success, which was reflected in the organization of the first congress on climatotherapy in Nice, in 1904.

Bathing in the air and sun implies exposing the skin, which is not without offence in France where nude sunbathing, alone or in groups, is much less welcomed than in Germany. Across the Rhine, a significant network of associations has developed to support these practices, which are considered by many to be non-conformist. On the eve of World War I, the *Naturheilvereine* had nearly 900,000 members across 900 local groups. Thereafter, the interwar period saw the development of naturist leisure practices promoted by the supporters of alternative ways of life, combined with other practices linked with "self-care", involving food practices (vegetarianism) but also alcoholic and tobacco abstinence and the practice of physical culture. In France, naturist leisure resorts have been created, such as *Physiopolis*, a naturist city of 16 hectares on the outskirts of Paris, which accommodates up to 2,000 visitors on sunny days with a slogan: "Here is beauty, here is health, here is peace" (Bauberot 2008). Naturism was promoted by doctors who, at the time, argued the curative power of nature, which they believed was preferable to many remedies from traditional pharmacopoeia. Contact between the body and the elements was considered as a way to strengthen the natural resistance of the organism to diseases.

The ideal conveyed at that time by naturism was also aesthetic and moral (being accustomed to nudity means that it should no longer be subject to depravity) in addition to being sanitary. Nudity was seen as a source "of blooming of the physical faculties and health conservation" (Bauberot 2008). While the naturist movements remained relatively marginal in terms of followers, they would have participated in the evolution of body norms.

The gradual shift from a medical to hedonistic approach continued during the second half of the 20th century with the development of coastal tourism, which continued to modify how the body was viewed. In a biomedical vision, the body is the carnal envelope of the individual. It clearly belongs to the private sphere and its care is a matter for a singular conversation between a caregiver and their patient. In a more hedonistic vision, the body is displayed and made visible: it becomes social. This transition was not radical but progressive and would gradually enhance practices such as tanning, which became fashionable after World War II and spread as a standard for beauty, especially for women, through magazines such as *Marie-Claire* and *Elle* (Ory 2008), in which blushers and whitening products were replaced by the promotion of suntan lotions and self-tanners. Fashion made tanning chic and the recently introduced paid vacations made it more democratic. Thus, for a few decades, sunbathing was no longer therapeutic but had a dual hedonic and aesthetic function, at least in the west, since, as we will see, body norms were subject to geographical variations. Coeffé et al. (2012) have shown, for example, how the figure of the Hawaiian surfer, tanned and muscular, has contributed to the enhancement of this image.

It is from the observation of a tripling of the cases of cutaneous cancers that the discourse on the exposing of bodies to the sun will take on a medical dimension. Studies show the relationship between too much exposure to ultraviolet rays and the occurrence of skin cancers (basal cell carcinoma, epidermoid carcinoma and melanoma) (Belot et al. 2008). The sun has been classified as a human carcinogen since 1992.

Tanning is now characterized by a contradiction. It continues to be valued aesthetically, and a tanned skin is still associated, in the western imagination, with good health. It is also true, as previously stated, that moderate exposure has positive effects such as promoting the synthesis of vitamin D, necessary for the absorption of calcium in the bones. However, for fair skin, exposure of 5–10 minutes, two to three times a week in summer, is sufficient to synthesize the maximum necessary quantity of the so-called "reserve" form of vitamin D: previtamin D3. Beyond this, previtamin D3 is destroyed by a self-regulatory mechanism to avoid any toxicity linked to an overdose. This is a far cry from the exposure times that can be observed in many tourist resorts. Conversely, the sun's ultraviolet (UVA and UVB) rays have harmful effects on health at high doses (Table 2.3): they damage DNA, cause skin aging, increase the risk of cancer, weaken the immune system and can lead to cataracts. The use of artificial tanning devices exacerbates these phenomena.

	UVB	**Sun**	**UVA**	**Artificial tanning**
Production of vitamin D	Yes	Yes	Low	Low
"Tanning" with protective effect	Yes	Yes	Low	Low
Immediate skin pigmentation	No	Yes	Yes	Yes
Sunburn	Yes	Yes	Low	Low
DNA damage	Yes	Yes	Yes	Yes
Cancers	Yes	Yes	Yes	Yes
Skin aging	Yes	Yes	Yes	Yes
Risk to eyes (cataracts, etc.)	Yes	Yes	Yes	Yes
Weakening of the immune system and inflammation	Yes	Yes	Yes	Yes

Table 2.3. *The main biological effects of UVB, sunlight, UVA and artificial UV tanning (source: INCA 2010)*

The WHO has published recommendations for tourism professionals regarding this risk, which is often neglected or obscured by aesthetic norms. These recommendations are made at several levels: globally, the INTERSUN program was launched in 1993 (Box 2.1.). It aims to reduce UV exposure by disseminating information and preventive recommendations. For example, it is in the wake of this program that the UV index has become widely used as a tool to raise awareness of the need for sun protection. This index has now entered into the mainstream in western societies, where people are used to seeing a UV index displayed during summer weather reports, as well as the presence of this index on the packaging of suntan lotions.

To provide information, practical advice and sound scientific predictions on the health impact and environmental effects of UV exposure.

To encourage countries to take action to reduce UV-induced health risks.

To provide guidance to national authorities and other agencies about effective sun awareness programs.

Box 2.1. *INTERSUN objectives (source: WHO, https://www.who.int/initiatives/intersun-programme/)*

At a more individual level, the WHO has published recommendations for the tourism industry to adopt virtuous behavior in the face of the risks associated with sun exposure and to inform their clients about their leisure activities at the local level (Box 2.2.). The argument developed for tour operators[24] is largely based on the comfort and pleasure of the tourist: "When the client falls ill or experiences pain, his ability to enjoy and participate in an activity is considerably diminished. This not only means an unhappy customer, but also a decrease in potential revenue for the tour operator. Unfortunately, many tourists also get sunburned, which in some cases can be severe, resulting from overexposure to the sun's ultraviolet rays." Consequently, the WHO recommends that tourism professionals develop information for their customers: before departure, by encouraging them to include hats, sunscreen and sunglasses in their luggage, and during their stay, to display prevention messages in different languages (the WHO offers documents and illustrations, including basic advice, translated into various languages). For example, tourists should be advised to wear covering clothing, which is often contrary to their desire to expose their skin to the sun as much as possible, in a bathing suit, in order to get a tan. While it is difficult to go against the tourists' wishes, even though they are harmful to themselves, it is possible, and even recommended, to organize activities and excursions so that tourists have access to shaded areas. Activities that involve long periods of exposure (such as sea outings, surface snorkeling, hiking and so on) should be scheduled during the hours of least solar radiation (avoiding the meridian hours of the day). In hotels and resorts, it is recommended to provide

24 https://www.who.int/uv/publications/en/touroperators.pdf, accessed 04/20/2020.

guests with sun protection (sun creams, hats, umbrellas and so on), whether free of charge or not.

> While customers are under your care … Special recommendations on what you can do.
>
> For excursion providers:
>
> – ensure sunscreen, sunglasses and hats are either freely available or for sale;
>
> – provide regular reminders to your customers of the importance to take precautions to prevent sunburn;
>
> – if customers are going to be left at any one place for a long time, ensure locations are chosen that have access to shade;
>
> – where shade does not exist, avoid leaving your customers for long periods exposed to the sun over the period of solar noon when the UV radiation is at its most intense. Instead plan the schedule so that long periods outdoors are at times when ultraviolet radiation levels are significantly lower, such as early morning or late in the afternoon.
>
> For resort managers – water based:
>
> – ensure sunscreen, sunglasses and hats are either freely available or for sale;
>
> – provide regular reminders to your customers of the importance to take precautions to prevent sunburn, especially on their arrival. Strategic use of signs to encourage sun protective behavior is encouraged;
>
> – ensure your facility has plenty of shade where customers are likely to congregate;
>
> – provide or rent beach umbrellas for customers if they do not already exist;
>
> – schedule events that may require long periods in direct sunlight away from peak UV periods. Instead plan the schedule in the early morning or late in the afternoon when the UV is significantly less intense.
>
> For resort managers – in mountain areas:
>
> – ensure sunscreen and sunglasses are available for sale;
>
> – provide regular reminders to your customers of the importance to take precautions to prevent sunburn and eye damage.

Box 2.2. *Guidelines for tour operators: minimizing the risks associated with UV exposure (source: WHO brochure)*

Recently, the problem of protection against solar radiation has become more complex since development of knowledge on the subject has shown that the use of sunscreens, protective for individuals, can present a serious risk of damaging the marine environment. Hundreds of millions of tourists visit the world's coasts every year and the sunscreen creams they apply to their skin on the beach end up largely diluted in the seas and oceans as they swim. Depending on the source, it is estimated that, every year, 15–25 million tons of sunscreen are thus spilled into marine waters. These creams contain titanium dioxide and zinc oxide compounds, particularly in the form of nanoparticles, which are toxic for marine ecosystems. These nanoparticles are extremely fine and can penetrate living organisms and disrupt them. Coral reefs, already largely impacted by climate change, are the first visible victims of this pollution. Phytoplankton is also strongly impacted, yet it is one of the main consumers of CO_2 and producer of oxygen. The ecological stakes are therefore high. Recently, a gradual awareness of this problem has been taking place. Some destinations prohibit the use of sunscreen during aquatic activities (this is the case, for example, in the lagoons of Hawaii or in certain diving sites on the Riviera Maya). Some manufacturers have put organic sunscreens reputed to be non-polluting (or, at least, less polluting) on the market, but these products are expensive and are not available in all sales outlets. It is however urgent that behaviors evolve so that the protection of health from solar radiation does not become harmful through the negative impact it would have on ecosystems. Coastal tourism must question its practices and customs and perhaps it is time that tanning, like other harmful trends, loses its appeal in order to limit its negative indirect effects. In some countries, moreover, the positive vision of tanning is not self-evident. The study "Tanning in China", conducted at the University of Angers in France, is not related to the ecological issue, but is nevertheless very interesting because of the social issues it raises, based on the assumption that the skin, the visible part of the body "allows us to communicate with the outside world not only by touch, but also by the image it conveys, so that it exposes us to the gaze of others. The skin is then a marker of historically built social and cultural standards" (Coëffé et al. 2019). Based on observations made on the island of Hainan (South China), a tourist destination frequented mainly by Chinese, the authors observed that the recent development of coastal tourism calls into question the "dominant aesthetic convention in China, which is that of a white, milky skin associated with the idea of purity". By exposing their bodies to tanning, Chinese tourists are effecting a form of transgression. However, this remains limited, as very few Chinese people allow themselves to lie on the beach and sunbathe for long periods of time, as westerners do. Also, while many men expose their bodies to the sun, women are reluctant, which is certainly related to social norms. Generally, they wear covering clothes or even a specific accessory: the "facekini", an invention initially intended to protect the face from jellyfish stings and which is also used to swim without tanning.

2.3.2. *Worship of bodily beauty*

Tanning, as mentioned above, is primarily for aesthetic reasons. Tourism has many other ways of taking care of the body through different practices. In a simplified way, we could place tourism and thus vacationing in opposition to work from the body point of view. While work alienates the body, tourism offers it freedom, takes it out of its routine and participates in a process of re-creation. Coëffé et al. (2016) evoke the (complementary) "four bodies" of the tourist. The first is the rested body, which takes advantage of the idleness of vacations and extracts itself from the rhythm of work. The second is the transformed body, which will, for example, allow itself to wear light clothing that it would not wear in the city, or even to strip off. The third is the body engaged through sports practices of varying intensity (walking, trekking, surfing and so on), which again constitute an "out of the ordinary" for individuals who are often sedentary the rest of the time. This engagement of the body is often accompanied by a quest for pleasure, the body rewarding this engagement through the secretion of endorphins. Finally, the fourth body of the tourist is called the "body to body" by the authors, and refers to encounters that often punctuate the tourist experience, as previously mentioned.

In the following sections, we develop some illustrations of the link between health, well-being of the body and tourism through sports activities, relaxation practices (such as massages) and, finally, some particular artifacts: tattoos, as painted in any one of the many tattoo studios that have been flourishing for a few years in tourist destinations.

2.3.2.1. *Sports, tourism and health*

Tourist trips are conducive to sports activities. Very often, vacations are an opportunity to try a sport related to the place where you are staying (water sports or mountaineering, for example). Sometimes, it is simply a time to break away from a "subway-work-sleep" rhythm that leaves little room for physical activity, as Noël Hureaux (2012) shows, using the example of walking. This activity, accessible to the vast majority of people regardless of their physical condition, is particularly simple, "consisting of taking a walk in order to find well-being". Strolling differs from hiking, which implies a more significant and prolonged effort. There are indeed various degrees of engagement of the body[25] in physical activity but, whatever the level, through walking, a bodily contact with a site, discovery and curious exploration takes place and enables something to be learned through mediation of the body (Brougère 2015).

The basis of the relationship between sports, tourism and health is the idea of being oxygenated and of breathing pure air (arguments often put forward in tourist communications). Bathing in the context of coastal tourism is based on the same idea: we take a dip without actually "swimming".

---

25 Here we adopt one of the categories suggested by Coëffé *et al.* (2016).

However, there are also sports activities associated with tourism that are similar to a real sporting effort, even a performance. Alpine skiing, for example, requires significant muscular and articular effort. However, very often, winter tourists arrive in the mountains having not trained beforehand, with a certain level of muscular preparation, and many do not warm up before taking their first ski lift. This explains a large proportion of the accidents recorded on ski slopes: sprains, fractures and various traumas related to falls. We also observe a variation in the frequency of these accidents depending on the time of day. Many falls with injuries occur due to accumulated fatigue, combined with lack of physical conditioning in individuals who are not athletic the rest of the year. A well-known insurance company warns on its website: "Physical and muscular fatigue appears after a few days of activity and mainly affects athletes who are not sufficiently prepared." Other risks not related to falls exist in skiing, as in many other sports, such as muscle injuries and tendinopathies.

Skiing is one example, but the list of sports offered in tourist destinations is long (climbing, trekking, mountain biking, tree climbing, rafting, kayaking, sailing, surfing, diving, golf and others) and physical activity is used to reinforce the attractiveness of destinations. According to Desmond (1999), it is even more profoundly a question of directing bodies: their appearance, their activities, where they practice and who sees them and so on. In her view, "the fantastic spectacle of physicality" forms the basis of a very profitable tourism industry that both exploits and structures identities and affiliations. The author bases her reasoning on the observation of surfers in Waikiki (Hawaii) and the way this group of sports tourists conveys an image and representations around the world that is similar to a (more or less idealized) way of life. This way of life includes considerations related to health: the body is shaped by sporting activity and by a healthy diet, the skin is tanned and so on. It is interesting to read interviews with Chinese surfers who have to deal with two cultural influences: that of their country, where whiteness is a beauty norm, and that of their sporting community, in which being white means that they would not have been surfing long enough to have been able to tan.

Tourism operators rarely bother with these nuances and put forward the fact of self-care through physical activity as an argument for attractiveness. While the playful aspect of these activities is undeniable (we also speak of "edutainment activities" – Bodin et al. 2009), in the background we also find a discourse globally conveyed by public health organizations at all levels, advocating an active lifestyle favorable to health at all ages. The French Academy of Medicine, for example, cites the prevention of being overweight or obesity in adolescents or the improvement of functional capacities in the elderly, which acts on numerous risk factors (in particular, cardiovascular), leading to a better quality of life for the elderly and delaying their entry into dependence (Pène and Touitou 2009). This document also underlines "the benefit of physical and sports activities in the primary prevention of many diseases, including cardiovascular and respiratory diseases, various bone loss syndromes, osteoporosis, metabolic diseases (obesity and type 2 diabetes) and breast and colon cancers, in particular, as well as its beneficial effect on psychological balance. Some countries, such as Germany, recognize the usefulness of prescribing physical and sporting activity for primary and secondary prevention of many diseases and have therefore included it in the list of services that are eligible for reimbursement by the health insurance system"[26].

Sports activities related to well-being and "self-care" are now a competitive factor for many tourist destinations. In 2014, the French national statistical and economic studies institute, INSEE, estimated that sports tourism represented nearly 12% of the country's tourism revenue. In a recent study (2015), Bouhaouala and Biard analyzed this phenomenon based on the French case of Vichy-Val d'Allier (VVA), which positions itself around a "year-round well-being and sports tourism" offer. In addition to thermalism, which is the region's main tourist attraction, the use of sports "becomes a card to play for VVA. Indeed, it participates in the tourism offer, meets the needs of residents and legitimizes public investment". One sport that is accessible to all physical levels stands out: golf. According to the above-mentioned authors, the impact of "golf tourism" constitutes between 20 and 90% of the turnover of 276 clubs in France and represents an investment with a high return in terms of tourist appeal. However, it is a significant investment and the triptych of sports-tourism-health must be approached with the principal idea of a gradient in amenities: walking and individual sports activities in nature require little infrastructure (e.g. a well-maintained hiking trail), whereas more demanding edutainment activities require heavy infrastructure (e.g. a water sports center) and trained and competent staff, particularly to prevent the risk of accidents (see below).

2.3.2.2. *Massages and other practices reinvented in tourist locations*

Another way to enjoy a tourist stay through the mediation of the body is the recourse to body care, at the forefront of which is massage, which some destinations have made a specialty (such as Bali or Thailand in Southeast Asia). Here, we return to the "body to body" evoked by Coëffé et al. where the tourist is "pampered" by a carnal contact that is something other than a sexual relationship. What happens in this process passes beyond the biomedical dimension of health, as Planelles (2018) points out in an analysis of tourism promotion discourses: "'Need to be pampered, to fill up on trace elements?' The term trace elements, which is a chemical term, plays a referential role. However, if we analyze the rest of the text, 'choose the Privilege fitness center with a massage every day', and the following photo of a handsome, relaxed man in the middle of a massage, we note that, in this case, in addition to the

26 http://www.senat.fr/lc/lc288/lc2881.html. Comparative Legislation Study No. 288, July 2019, collection of briefing notes from March to June 2019: medically prescribing physical activity for some therapeutic purposes, accessed 04/22/2020.

referential function, it is the evocative function of quality of life and health that the receiver activates in the context of an advertisement, for which a knowledge of chemistry is not necessary in order to understand the message."

What is happening around the offer of massages to tourists is particularly revealing of the link between tourism and health: both present and essential and, at the same time, set aside.

Let us take the example of a destination such as the island of Bali in Indonesia[27]. Its tourism development was certainly due to its beaches and landscapes and the waves of Kuta which attracted surfers from Australia and around the world. However, this tourism development was also based on an image of well-being and holistic health specific to the Balinese culture and which can be summarized by the term *Tri Hita Karana*. This is a Balinese holism that is much less studied than the Indian Ayurveda (see, for example, Sathyanarayana and Snehalatha 2011) and which links the health of the body to the health of the mind and the environment: in a way, the premises of sustainable development! For the Balinese, a disease that can be treated by doctors is one that depends on the relationship between humans and nature. The unbalanced acts depend on other traditional healers and if the imbalance is in the relationship between humans and God, then the treatment is spiritual. Thus, for the Balinese, health is in the spiritualism (body and soul). There are many purification and meditation ceremonies for healing, which are related to health but are not displayed as health, rather as culture and belief. For example, going to the temple or to the beach can be experienced as healing for a Balinese.

Some tourists seek to learn about these practices in varying degrees (from visiting temples, to participating in purification ceremonies, to consulting *balians*, traditional healers). However, this spiritual health tourism is not a commercial attraction and practicing this kind of tourism is a proactive approach and a real search for information off the beaten track. Yet, during in-depth discussions with Balinese, there is a sense of aspiration to emphasize these cultural aspects of health rather than to conform to the aspirations of mass tourism, which involves distorting the traditional vision to adapt it to western tourists. From then on, massage appears to be a very good way to mediate between the tourist's aspirations and the idea of monetizing a piece of local culture as a tourist experience.

Massages are offered everywhere in Bali: on the beach, in the shopping streets and so on, with no real thought to care, other than well-being or relaxation (Figure 2.14). This is a misappropriation of cultural heritage that has become a

27 The following remarks have already been published in a similar form by the author of this book, in an article published in the journal *Carnets de Géographes* in 2020.

tourism marketing product. Few masseuses are trained[28]: in spas, masseuses report three months of "informal" training, while the majority of on-beach massage practitioners are self-taught.

However, massage is a traditional care gesture in Bali that has developed in a direction of relaxation for tourists. In the local culture, it is more a care of the spirit as one Balinese woman confided to us during a field trip to this island: "There is a base of Balinese culture around health traditions. So when we think about business development, we think about how to relax the tourist." Traditional Balinese wisdom proposes massages requiring more extensive non-conventional training and the use of *bokashi* essential oils (or lemon to remove toxins from the skin). Some villages are developing a community tourism in which tourists are invited to discover the Balinese way of life. Several villages have formed associations, none of which has chosen to offer *jamu* (herbal preparations) and *boreh* (wraps with traditional ointments and massages with coconut oil). The use of health as a tourist attraction is not based on the modern vision of health but on a more spiritual vision: the tourist is initiated to take care of their body and their mind.

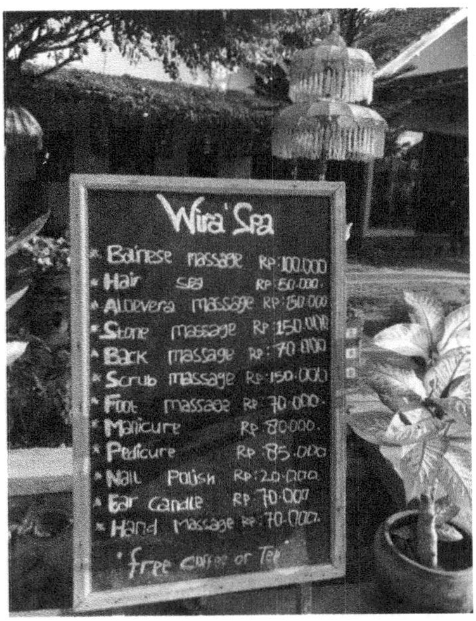
Wira Spa
Bainese massage RP 100.000
Hair spa RP 50.000
Aloevera massage RP 150.000
Stone massage RP 150.000
Back massage RP 70.000
Scrub massage RP 150.000
Foot massage RP 70.000
Manicure RP 80.000
Pedicure RP 85.000
Nail Polish RP 20.000
Ear Candle RP 70.000
Hand massage RP 70.000
free coffee or Tee

Figure 2.14. *Rates for wellness services in a spa in Bali (photo: S. Fleuret 2016)*

28 This profession is predominantly female.

Spirituality, massage and food (which we have not mentioned but which is also important in Bali) are the pillars of a health tourism which dares not speak its name, however, without any real training and without any real connection between traditional medicine and a recreational offering.

Sales of traditional massage oils and herbal preparations remain relatively marginal in Bali, but other tourist destinations have taken advantage of these types of products to combine the sale of local, traditional products with tourism, which provides the bulk of the clientele, all supported by a sales pitch related to body care. Morocco is an excellent example with its exploitation of argan oil.

In the south west of Morocco, in a triangle connecting Essaouira, Tiznit and Taroudant, is the world's only endemic area for the argan tree, a shrub whose fruit is used to produce argan oil. It takes time and more than 30 kilos of fruit to produce this oil, which, in addition to its culinary virtues, is used in cosmetics and as a miraculous remedy for many ailments. Argan oil is reputed to reduce the risk of cardiovascular disease and the effects of aging. It is also used against burns, dermatitis, rheumatism, for daily skin and hair care.

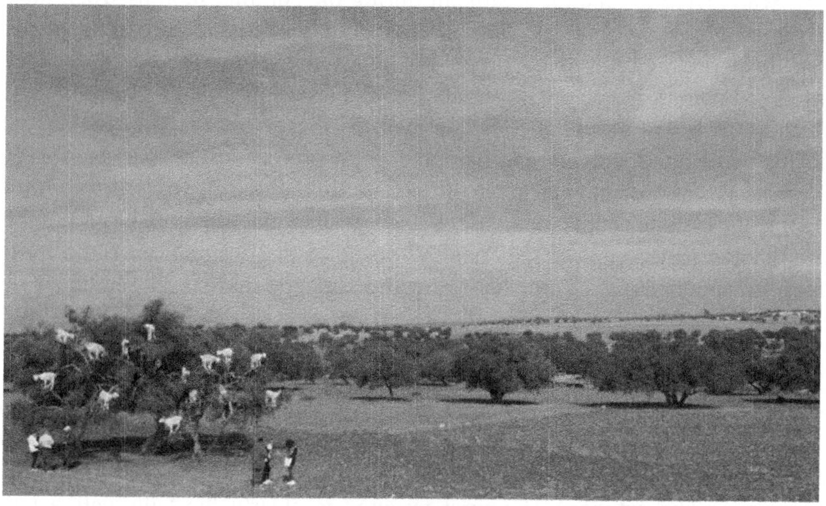

Figure 2.15. *Argan trees between Marrakech and Essaouira in Morocco (photo: S. Fleuret 2017)*

Given the difficulty of producing this oil, its profitability was, for a time, called into question. Its production is ensured essentially by Berber women from the villages of the region. To ensure their economic survival, they began, in the 1990s, to form cooperatives, which enabled them to improve their living conditions in these very rural and arid areas (Figure 2.15). Soon, tourists to the region proved to be an excellent outlet for the products of these communities, such as edible oil, *amlou* (a spread said to be an aphrodisiac) and various cosmetics (such as soaps and creams). These products have spread to the tourist resorts and have become some of the brand images of southern Morocco, which some unscrupulously exploit in resorts which are cooperatives in name only and which sell low quality cut oil and industrial cosmetics to busloads of tourists.

Other attempts have been made to exploit the natural resources of the region based on the same agenda related to health and well-being. This is the case at the margins of the Sahara with the development of sand baths (Gélard 2014), which involve being buried in hot sand (70–80°C), enabling excess moisture contained in the body to be absorbed into the bones and thus heal joint pain, especially rheumatism. This is an age-old practice: the Tuaregs would have typically used the heat of the sand (naturally or by heating it) to relieve their lumbar pains. A neologism accompanies these practices, which seem to have been in full expansion since the end of the 1980s: sand therapy. The region of Merzouga in Morocco has recently become a well-known sand therapy destination and attracts mainly elderly people living in the north of the country, who arrive to take the treatment during the summer months when the sand is at its hottest[29]. According to Gélard (2014), "the desert is thought of as the perfect place to heal bodies bruised by urban life (caused by humidity of coastal cities, pollution and so on), hence the importance of the desert as a place of healing". Once again, it is medical tourism that will transform these resorts. This region, which previously welcomed only a small number of visitors, desert tourists, for tented experiences, is now urbanizing to accommodate this new influx of visitors, through developments of hotel capacities, stores and services, including a large number of herbalist stores that complete the "health" decor of the destination. Little by little, national therapeutic tourists are replacing the western tourists in search of desert discovery.

On the other side of the Atlantic, on the Riviera Maya in Mexico, we can also see the reuse of an age-old care technique, the *temazcal*, in an attempt to develop a different well-being and health tourism from the mass tourism that is observed in Cancún. For the Mayan communities, the challenge is to glean benefits from the tourist manna. The category of tourist targeted is clearly the "alternative tourist" (Neyra 2019), in search of an "authentic" experience and a reconnection with nature and local history.

29 The practice of burial in hot sand is not without risk and many cases of discomfort have occurred, leading to a reorganization of the practice, notably by limiting the time spent buried. However, the practice remains poorly supervised and anyone can become an expert in sand therapy.

The word *temazcal* comes from the Náhuatl language and literally means "house of hot stones", effectively a sweat lodge in which steam is produced by pouring water over heated stones. These sweating practices are widespread in almost all Amerindian territories. Similar to the sauna, or hammam, it is a relaxation space in which steam is used to eliminate toxins. The function of the *temazcal* is at the same time curative, social and also spiritual: to relax the body and the mind.

Temazcal is today put forward in the tourist offer in the Yucatán Peninsula in Mexico, to complement the classic spa offering. The Mayan thread is exploited for its "neo-traditional" connotation in the spirit of a tourism that seeks to be an "authentic" experience. For all that, the traditional Mayan massages offered in wellness salons in the hotels or streets of Cancún, Playa del Carmen or Tulum, are only Mayan in name. During fieldwork, we asked the masseurs who offered them what they were and what traditional knowledge they were based on, and the answers were: "It's like a classic massage, but more expensive" and "I don't know, I was told it was traditional, but I don't know exactly what knowledge it refers to." Indeed, on researching scientific literature to learn more about these famous traditional Mayan massages, it transpires that only the massages of young pre- and post-natal women are documented as traditional Mayan massage practices (Folliard 2008). We will return to the instrumentalization of traditional health knowledge as a tourism marketing tool later in this book.

A final example can be developed to illustrate "self-care" practices during tourist stays: the relatively new offering of "health packages" of different levels of specialization, where the tourist buys a stay that includes discovering a resort with accommodation and a more or less specialized offer of services related to health. For example, near Agadir in Morocco, you can spend a week in a guest house in the hinterland, in a quiet place far from the tourist flow, for a stay combining nutritherapy (adapted meals with the objective of losing weight), physical activity (hiking) and relaxation and meditation sessions. The owner of the guest house offering this type of stay is also a nutritionist doctor in the neighboring town. His argument to convince tourists is reflected in the slogan: "Take advantage of your vacation to reclaim your body."

2.3.2.3. *Getting a tattoo on vacation, attractions and inconveniences*

There is another practice that is currently very successful, linked to transforming the body in the typology proposed by Coëffé et al. which consists of getting a tattoo during a tourist stay, as a souvenir to bring home from a trip. In many destinations, tattoo parlors are open day and night, as illustrated by the photos in Figure 2.16, taken in Khaosan Road, Bangkok, Thailand. They engrave bodies with indelible ink, for the more daring, while small shops offer temporary tattoos that fade in a few days. These practices are not harmless or without risks.

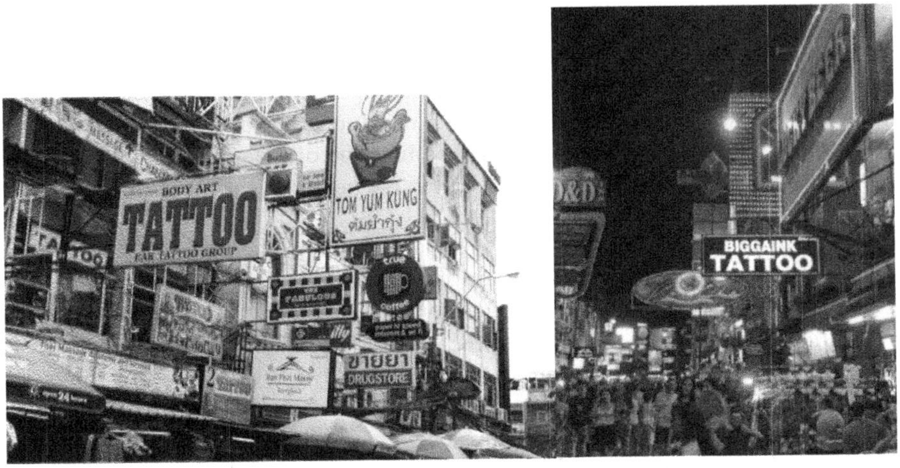

Figure 2.16. *Khaosan Road, Bangkok, Thailand (photos: S. Fleuret 2016)*

Tattooing and travel have a long history together. For a long time, tattooed bodies have been those from well-identified categories of the population: remote tribes (such as the Polynesians and Maoris) and "tough guys", sailors (then convicts) with very distinct iconographies. In both cases, tattoos convey elements of social and cultural identity as well as well-established codes conveyed by the bodies of migrants or travelers returning from exotic destinations (Cohen 2013).

Since the beginning of the 2000s, the practice of tattooing has been democratized, and it is estimated today that nearly a third of the western population aged under 30 has tattoos. This democratization has been accompanied by a dilution of the meaning and scope of tattooed symbols and motifs. While the tribal tattoo remains one of the most common motifs, it is chosen more for the aestheticism of its graphics than for its identity or spiritual meaning. In the societies of Oceania, tattoos accompany rites of passage: this is the case in Samoa for example, where the *pe'a* (male tattoo) was necessary to obtain a wife and marked belonging to the village force (*malosi o le nu'u*) and the group of young men (*taulele'a*) in charge of serving and protecting the chieftaincy. Today, in Samoa, the tattoo remains a sign of allegiance to the group of chiefs (*matai*) and signals respect for their authority (Galliot 2009). Although it can be extrapolated that getting a tattoo while traveling may also be a rite of passage[30], westerners who wear such a tattoo are very often unaware of its deeper meaning. However, some authors believe that tattooing may be becoming a constituent element of travel culture (Cohen 2013). In Polynesia, tattooing is one of the vectors for

30 It was common for sailors to get tattoos when crossing the equator in times when crossing this imaginary line was not as common as it is nowadays.

promoting cultural tourism and, according to Ginolin (2004), we are witnessing "a specialization of artisanal productions in the archipelagos [which] contributes to the affirmation of local cultural specificity, following, in particular, the example of the Marquesas Islands, which for the past twenty years, have been asserting the originality of their culture through the valorization of their sculptures, *tapa* or contemporary tattoos". This phenomenon responds to a "tourist demand for a reinterpreted pre-European artisanal heritage".

In tourist destinations, tattoo parlors offer designs that have very little to do with existing local tattoo culture. Certainly in Bangkok, Auckland or Tahiti you can get a traditional tattoo, sometimes using a traditional technique (such as bamboo sticks or bones). However, most of the time, the proposed designs are standardized and can be found anywhere, whatever the destination, just like the handmade souvenirs *made in China*.

Seen through the prism of health, this phenomenon raises several questions. Tattooing is not a practice without risks. First, introducing a needle under the skin carries risks of infection and transmission of diseases (HIV-AIDS, hepatitis and so on), which raises the question of the hygiene of the tattoo parlors and its control by the authorities[31]. In France, a hygiene charter has established material hygiene and sterilization rules since 2003. It was put together by the *Syndicat National des Artistes Tatoueurs* (National Union of Tattoo Artists) and by doctors. Moreover, compulsory theoretical training in hygiene is a legal requirement. Tattooing must be carried out using a dermograph (an electric tattooing machine), single-use or sterilized needles, wearing gloves and using dyes, for which the composition must be provided by the manufacturer[32].

Once the tattoo has been safely completed, the healing phase begins, and in this case, getting a tattoo during a tourist stay may not be a good idea, especially if you wait until the last day of your stay to have it done. Indeed, sun, bathing and salt are enemies of healing. Someone who gets a tattoo in Playa del Carmen or by the beach in Phuket, for example, should not expose themselves to the sun or swim, either in the sea or in the hotel pool, which is paradoxical considering that these are the main attractions of these sea, sand and sun destinations.

There are two types of risk: aesthetic and sanitary. Aesthetically, the sun and water (especially sea water) will have a blotting effect that will diffuse the ink under the skin and make the lines "smudge", causing the design to be less clear and even

31 Europe, France or the United States, for example, have strict regulations concerning tattooing hygiene and ink quality, but there is not, to our knowledge, a list and even less a cartography of countries at risk concerning the practice of permanent tattooing.
32 Source: http://www.dermagazine.fr/tatouages-quels-risques/.

irredeemably unattractive. Exposure to the sun will also have the effect of dulling the colors.

From the sanitary perspective, skin is not naturally adapted to tattooing, which opens a breach in the cutaneous barrier and causes the rupture of many small vessels of the skin. This constitutes an entry point for infectious agents (e.g. staphylococci or mycobacteria), and thus necessitates regular disinfection of the wounds during the whole period of cicatrization (around 10 days minimum). Swimming is a risk factor since water contains many germs that are potentially infectious for a wound. In addition, the insertion of foreign bodies (colored pigments) under the skin may be accompanied by an inflammatory reaction as the organism tries to reject these colorants, which it considers to be intruders. A mild reaction is normal, but in some cases, chronic inflammation can occur, causing tissue necrosis. Other allergic-type reactions can occur: reactions to products contained in the inks and the traceability requirements imposed on manufacturers in countries with legislation generally enables identification of, and treatment for, allergic sensitivity. This is not the case for the "beach" tattooers in countries less focused on hygiene standards, who are not subject to such vigilance.

The sanitary risks also concern another practice frequently associated with tattooing: piercing, which consists of puncturing the skin in order to insert a piece of jewelry. The most frequent problem is the occurrence of allergies to nickel, the metal contained in the jewelry affixed during the piercing.

Some tourists try less definitive activities that do not involve intradermal lesions, such as henna tattooing. Several destinations, notably the Maghreb countries (including Morocco and Tunisia) or India, present this activity as a local cultural tourist experience, these tattoos being frequently worn as an ornament by local women for whom it is an attribute of seduction. The history is said to date back to the prophet Abraham: he had two wives, and his first wife was jealous of the second. To make her ugly and less desirable in the eyes of their husband, she regularly braided her co-wife's hair and drew henna patterns on her skin. However, contrary to her expectations, Abraham became more and more in love with his second wife, whom he found even more desirable due to her decoration. As well as a sign of seduction, the traditional henna tattoo is considered to be a protection against evil spirits. Through a wide variety of forms and symbols, it constitutes a veritable language largely watered down in a catalogue proposed to tourists in emblematic places like the Jemaa el-Fnaa square in Marrakech.

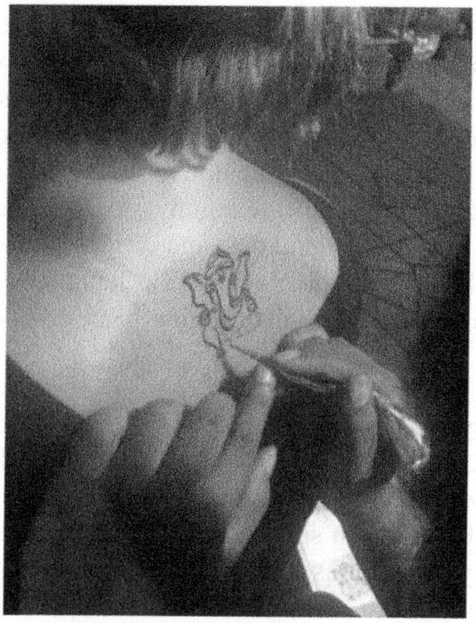

Figure 2.17. *Temporary black henna tattoo in a Bangkok street (photo: S. Fleuret 2016)*

However, here again, the activity involves risk because the tradition has been transformed in order to respond to the temporalities of tourism. Natural henna is brown in color, tending to red or orange, and requires a long application time (from 2 to 12 hours). However, tourists do not have this time available, especially since the application area must remain still during the drying of the henna. A substance is therefore added to the preparation, paraphenylenediamine (PPD), to reduce the application time and intensify the color, which then turns black (without PPD this depends on the drying time). This substance is responsible for numerous complications: localized contact eczema, sometimes secondarily generalized; scars resembling blisters and temporary or permanent pigmentary disorders; urticaria; angioedema; and anaphylactic shock (Le Coz 2001; Kluger et al. 2008). These reactions lead to allergic sensitization which can be combined with allergies to other substances, such as hair dyes or certain textile dyes. These consequences are therefore far from trivial and tourists should be wary of black henna tattoos (Figure 2.17), since international regulations are still not in place.

Finally, we must discuss the case of tourists who have been tattooed before their trip and who may be confronted with local contexts in which tattooing is very badly viewed, or even condemned by law. In several countries, tattooing is considered as a voluntary transformation of the body created by God and is therefore a blasphemy. For example, tourists visiting Dubai are advised to hide their tattoos.

On this subject, Japan is an eloquent case study, with its tradition of tattooing and even a style recognized around the world (*Iruzemi*). Historically, this style was prized by the nobility and later by a certain bourgeoisie as true works of art (an *Iruzemi* can still cost several tens of thousand Euros and require years of work). However, in Japan, tattooing generally had a poor image due to its use as a punishment to publicly mark bandits with a stigmatizing mark of infamy. As a consequence of this judicial marking, bandits tended to gather around this sign of recognition which has over time become a marker of belonging to the Yakuza (the Japanese mafia). The practice of tattooing was forbidden and therefore clandestine from 1870 until its legalization in 1948.

This historical and symbolic background is not without consequences for tattooed tourists who visit Japan. Indeed, many places have been forbidden to tattooed people, in particular the *Onsens*, the famous Japanese baths that are an important tourist attraction that can also be found in some hotels; however, the situation is changing. First, Japan is not totally impervious to the western trend of tattooing and increasing numbers of young Japanese are getting tattooed with patterns quite different from the traditional *Iruzemi* and which cannot be confused with Yakuza tattoos (which are small size realizations). Next, a tolerance is progressively developing towards tattooed foreigners (since foreign Yakuzas do not exist) and some *Onsens* are allowing them access (sometimes asking them to apply a temporary flesh-colored patch on their skin to hide the tattoos). Finally, in view of the organization of the 2020 Olympic Games, and in anticipation of an influx of western tourists and athletes (a number of them tattooed), the Japanese government addressed tourism professionals and the managers of public baths, to ask them for more tolerance and to open their baths and swimming pools to tattooed people. As it transpires, the Games were postponed to 2021 because of Covid-19, and, for the same reasons, it was considered probable that the influx of visitors would be less than expected. Nevertheless, the prospect of this event will have allowed tourism to contribute, albeit slowly in Japan, to an evolution in perceptions and body norms.

To conclude on the subject of tattoos, one study estimated that 50% of tattooed people regretted their tattoos (Burris and Kim 2007) and were possibly considering a laser erasure procedure, which is costly and not without risks, hence the common sense recommendation about thinking carefully before having a tattoo and to avoid getting one on impulse after a little too much to drink during a tourist stay. Unfortunately, there are too many anecdotes about such facts to relate them here.

2.4. Accidents, insurance and repatriation and access to travel healthcare

The 12 countries who are the main sources of tourists are divided between Europe (Germany, the United Kingdom, France, the Netherlands, Italy, Belgium and Spain), North America (the United States and Canada) and Asia (Japan, China and South Korea). They account for more than 50% of international tourist travel (Dehoorne et al. 2008) and all have health insurance systems that provide varying levels and types of coverage to their populations on a daily basis. However, the growth in the number of people going on overseas vacations sometimes means that coverage must be expanded to meet the needs of the traveler, since, in terms of health, during a trip abroad, travel or repatriation insurance can be useful in case of an urgent return.

Recent changes in the insurance sector have modified the organization of travel activity within those companies whose "travel" businesses have been affected by mergers involving the entire insurance world (Lohoré 2018). Numerous mergers have indeed taken place as part of a capitalist game that we do not detail here, but which has resulted in two distinct products: insurance and assistance, which are different and are therefore managed independently of each other. Assistance provides logistical support in the event of a problem during the tourist stay, while insurance provides compensation.

It should be noted here that care received overseas in the context of medical tourism, that is, travel abroad for therapeutic purposes, is not covered by this type of insurance.

The health safety of the tourist depends on the performance of the destination's health systems as well as on the insurance and assistance systems to which the tourist may have subscribed.

2.4.1. *Comparing healthcare systems around the world*

Traveling for tourist reasons, whatever the distance, means that, in case of need, recourse to a care service will be in an unfamiliar environment, with professionals or an organization of which the tourist knows little or nothing. However, there are significant geographical variations in the scope, nature and quality of the care offered from one country to another, and also within countries. Before a trip, it would be legitimate to ask the following question: is the healthcare system of the destination where I am about to go on vacation fit for purpose?

Reality tells us two things: first, the number of people who ask this question is surprisingly small. For example, we conducted two field surveys: one with tourists of all ages going to Agadir in Morocco and the other with elderly tourists on long stays (three weeks to three months) in Saly Portudal, in Senegal. In both cases, the majority of the people interviewed had not sought any information about the local healthcare system, considering that they were covered by their repatriation insurance[33]. Second, the question of the "performance" of health systems that condition the supply and availability of care is a subject that requires some clarification. This is the subject of the following section.

2.4.1.1. *Measuring the performance of a health system?*

In June 2000, the WHO published a ranking that assessed the health systems of its 191 member states on the basis of five performance indicators. The high-profile analysis concluded that France provided the best overall healthcare, followed by Italy, Spain, Oman, Austria and Japan. Following this publication, the numbers of international rankings have multiplied, with different indicators and methodologies that significantly vary the place of each country in the hierarchy. For example, the Bloomberg Healthiest Country Index, published in 2019, placed France in 12th place, but the criteria used in the study were quite different from those used by the WHO, making the two rankings difficult to compare.

Through these performance comparisons, what is sought to be highlighted is "the improvement in health status attributable to the healthcare system, the quality of care, the ability of the system to meet the expectations of populations, equity in access to care, and productive efficiency" (Paris 2012). It is important to keep in mind that there is no single measure of health system performance. These measures are the result of a combination of indicators, and changing even one of them can significantly alter the overall picture. Broadly speaking, these measures are

> On the one hand, health measures, primarily in the form of life event statistics, which provide information on the health status of the population. However, these indicators provide only a minor estimate of the impact of a health system on health status due to the role of other factors, such as human biology, lifestyle or environment. On the other hand, there are economic indicators that make it possible to evaluate efficiency (capacity to satisfy user demand and productivity) and equity (according to a priori defined principles of social justice). (Hartmann 2009)

33 This contributes to the idea that health is an afterthought of tourism, which is discussed in the last part of this book.

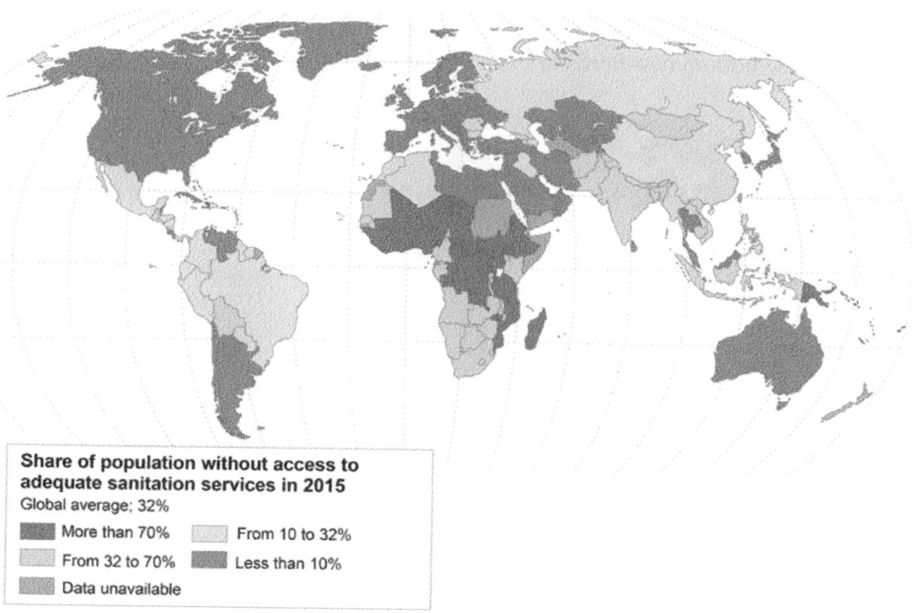

Figure 2.18. *Population without access to adequate sanitation (sources: World Health Organization and UNICEF, Progress on Sanitation and Drinking Water – 2015 update and MDG assessment; background map: FNSP. Sciences Po – Cartography workshop CC BY 4.0; design and production: Fleuret S., Lepetit A., UMR 6590 ESO)*

What interests us in any report on tourism and health is, first, the capacity of healthcare systems to take care of tourists in the event of an accident or illness during their stay and, second, the role that tourism development could have in structuring the supply of care. This second aspect is developed in Chapter 4 of this book, but Figure 2.18 is presented here because it provides an order of magnitude of the issues at stake: on average, nearly one-third of the world's population does not have access to adequate health services[34].

Figure 2.19 is ultimately more interesting than any ranking. It shows us that the world can be roughly divided into thirds according to the level of health performance of each country (here a UN study based on 33 indicators is used as a reference). Not surprisingly, western countries are in the most favored third and African countries in the most disadvantaged third. It is interesting to observe where the major international tourist destinations in the intertropical zone are located. With

34 The data used for this mapping predates the armed conflict in Libya. Today, the health situation in that country has deteriorated considerably and its political instability does not allow for reliable information to update this data.

the exception of a few destinations in the Gulf of Mexico and the Caribbean, most of them are in the bottom two-thirds or even the bottom third.

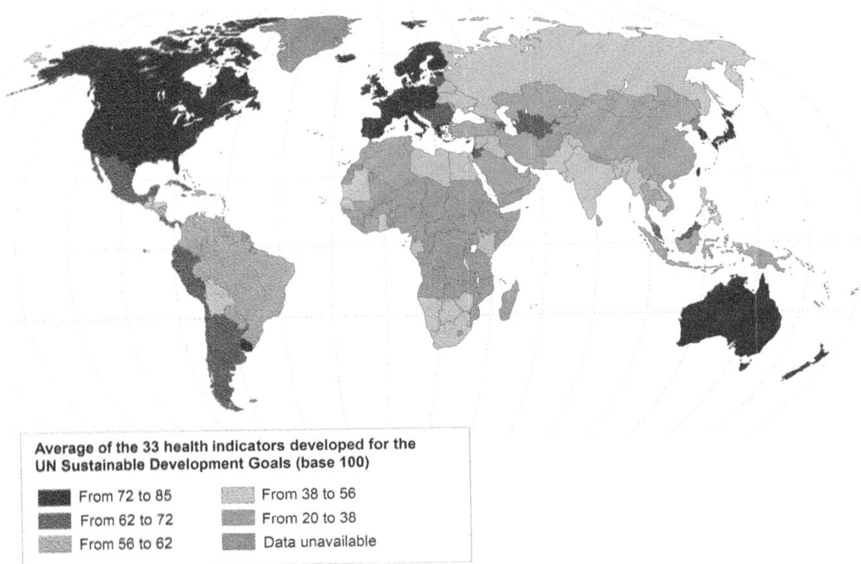

Figure 2.19. *Health performance around the world (source: GBD 2015 SDG Collaborators, Measuring the health-related Sustainable Development Goals in 188 countries: a baseline analysis from the Global Burden of Disease Study 2015, The Lancet, 2016; background map: FNSP. Sciences Po – Cartograhy workshop CC BY 4.0; design and production: Fleuret S., Lepetit A., UMR 6590 ESO)*

Thus, we should be able to distinguish safe destinations from a health point of view, that is, tourist destinations where, in the event of a health problem, the local system will be able to take care of tourists according to high-quality standards, equivalent to what they would find in countries with the most efficient healthcare systems. Other destinations, on the contrary, are not very safe in terms of healthcare.

This can be problematic. In order to understand this, we need to look at things in a little more detail, abandoning composite indicators and looking instead at specific indicators. Trauma is one of these explicit indicators, since trauma departments are where victims of road accidents, for example, are treated. However, there are countries that have only partial expertise in traumatology and very often these are the same countries that, as they lack a developed transport infrastructure, will make tourists travel in crowded vehicles with no safety standards or without helmets on motorcycle taxis, which are conducive to accidents and cranial, spinal and peripheral traumas. These injuries from accidents are sometimes fatal or, when they are not, can leave long-lasting consequences. One study found that people who suffer trauma (life-threatening) are six times more likely to die in low-income settings (36% mortality rate) than in high-income settings (6% mortality rate) (Mock et al. 2004). This is mainly due to difficulties in accessing hospitals (related to the quality of the road network, emergency transport services and so on), lack of equipment (such as respiratory assistance and CT scanners) and poor organization of healthcare services. This led the WHO to issue a practical guide for improving essential trauma care in 2004 (Mock et al. 2004), as these improvements can significantly reduce mortality and morbidity associated with trauma. Nevertheless, the shortcomings of some health systems make assistance and repatriation arrangements essential. Conversely, some destinations will concentrate services due to the very presence of tourists who make them necessary. This offer is sometimes subject to seasonal variations.

2.4.1.2. *Tourism, health and seasonality of supply*

Depending on the destination, the number of tourists may vary significantly according to the season, or even be completely seasonal, as is the case with ski resorts. In other destinations, although resorts are visited all year round by tourists, there may be peaks in visitor numbers at certain times (which often coincide with the vacation periods of the sending countries). This seasonality varies the supply of tourist services, and also affects the supply of healthcare: it is necessary to adapt the scope of the healthcare system to the volume of the population to be served, both the permanent and temporary population. A study published by the Auvergne-Rhône-Alpes regional health observatory (*Observatoire Régional de la Santé*, ORS) in France helps to illustrate this point (Fontaine et al. 2011).

This region is home to the world's leading ski resorts and is also a summer tourism destination, which makes it an area characterized by two tourist seasons, each marked by a temporary influx of population into communes that are sparsely populated during the rest of the year. The ORS study analyzed the activity of general practitioners based on health insurance data and shows "a winter peak accompanied by a high level of trauma activity". However, this seasonality varies from one commune to another. Some (the lowest number) have almost no activity off-season, but this becomes very high in winter, with a doubling of the number of general practitioners due to the arrival of seasonal doctors (15% of the doctors in the area studied have an exclusively seasonal practice). Other communes see an increase in healthcare activity during the winter sports season, which is maintained at a good level during the rest of the year, either thanks to a fairly large resident population or because the number of summer tourists is also fairly high. Finally, a third category of communes is less attractive in season (notably the small mid-mountain resorts), and as a result, there are no significant seasonal variations in healthcare activity. Across the whole of the tourist area studied, the year-round medical density is 11 general practitioners per 10,000 inhabitants. The influx of tourists in season is not compensated for by seasonal doctors – far from it – and the medical density is then halved (6 per

10,000). Doctors adapt to seasonality by increasing their practice opening hours or by only taking their vacations out of season. The season thus imposes on them, like other seasonal workers in the tourism industry, an intense rhythm over a given period. When asked about this, they see both advantages and disadvantages. In terms of advantages, the doctors cite the diversity of the practice and the benefits of a long off-season rest period. On the contrary, they cite some disadvantages, such as the significant investment costs they have to incur, because real estate is expensive in tourist areas and because they have to acquire expensive medical imaging equipment in order to diagnose traumas related to winter sports activities. Traumatology is a particularity that differentiates the practice of general medicine in winter sports resorts from the rest of the territory: it is relatively time-consuming and, as a result, the time devoted to treating these patients is time that is not available for the rest of the population. However, the patient base in these places also includes populations that may experience significant difficulties, such as seasonal workers who are often high-risk and subject to harmful working conditions (this point is developed in Chapter 4). Another group of the patient base, the year-round residents, is a rather aging population with health problems associated with age. As a result, some mid-mountain resorts may find themselves on the verge of a shortage of doctors, not in terms of medical density, but in terms of the available consultation time of the doctors present. The study by the Rhône-Alpes ORS concludes with a reflection on the location of medical practices. Should these be installed directly at the foot of the slopes so that they are more easily accessible to patients with trauma, or should they be located further downstream so that one practice can serve several resorts? This question is linked to another, the articulation of medical activity with that of tourism operators: should we organize the way in which operators are able to direct their clients towards the healthcare offer according to their needs and resources? Should they be asked to contribute to the additional health costs associated with tourism activities? The study does not answer these questions, which are still relevant today.

Another study (ORS Pays de la Loire 2008), conducted this time on a coastal tourist area, in the Vendée, attests to the seasonal variation in healthcare activity with other indicators. Activity at the control center, which receives medical emergency calls, increases by 43% during the months of July and August, and this is essentially reflected in the numbers of hospital cases. However, unlike in the mountain resorts, there is no increase in general practitioner activity in the Vendée during the summer: on the contrary, the average number of cases per doctor, expressed as an annual total, is 5,500 per year, with a peak of over 6,000 for January and February (linked to seasonal epidemics), with a dip in the summer (only 3,500 cases). This can be explained by several factors: first, the number of doctors increases slightly during the season, which distributes the activity among a greater number of practitioners and mechanically reduces the number of cases per individual. Second, coastal activities are less likely to cause physical injuries than winter sports. Finally, a large proportion of the situations requiring care are referred to health establishments closer to the seaside tourist areas than to the mountains. It is therefore in these establishments that the seasonal variation is felt. With regard to the emergency services, there is increased activity in the summer, with callouts 37% higher than in the rest of the year. The same report indicates that this seasonal variation is low in other hospital services (medicines, surgeries and obstetrics), attesting to a spike in activity linked to a "passing" patient population (the population of the Vendée department practically doubles in summer, from 580,000 to 1,120,000). The proportion of Vendée non-residents in hospital emergency room visits is 10% over the year and 35% during the summer months. All of this information is summarized in the graph in Figure 2.20.

Unfortunately, the study does not indicate whether the staffing levels of the departments affected by the seasonal surge in activity are reinforced by new recruits during the period in question, or whether this increase in activity results in an overload of work for the caregivers present all year round.

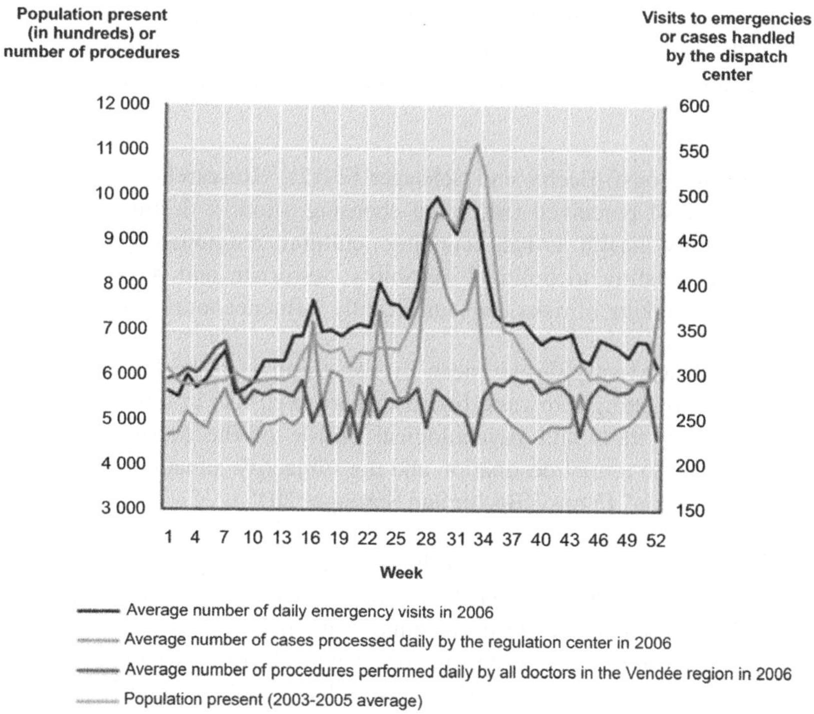

Figure 2.20. *Medical cases and emergency room activities according to the population present (source: estimate by the Tourism Department, the Vendée Control Center, Urcam-CPAM (excluding SLI, MSA and RSI), data transmitted by the participating health establishments, ORS exploitation)*

2.4.2. *Health insurance, assistance and repatriation*

While the hazards of life mean that health problems can occur even on vacation, a time when we should be leaving our worries behind, recourse to care does not necessarily happen at the place of the tourist stay and may require repatriation, maybe because the care offering in place is insufficient, or perhaps judged as being of lower quality than internationally accepted standards. This qualitative representation rarely comes from the tourists themselves, who do not ask for information on the health systems or on the healthcare offer. More often, it is the consular services of the sending countries, tourist guides and tour operators who alert travelers to possible risks and encourage them to take precautionary measures (pre-departure health check-ups, taking out insurance and so on).

2.4.2.1. *Perceived risk and behaviors*

As we have seen previously, the risk of accidents during travel is a function of the behavior of tourists confronted with an unfamiliar environment in which their points of reference become blurred, of their reduced vigilance during rest periods, and of the capacity of the various tourism operators to make their destinations more or less safe (Page and Meyer 1996). However, the perception and understanding of risk are highly subjective.

According to Yousfi-Bachir and Schaaper (2017), "Researchers have identified eight dimensions of perceived risk when choosing a tourist destination: terrorism, political instability, health, crime, economic, cultural, religious dogma and natural disasters. Risks relating to political instability, terrorism and physical health are assigned the top ranking of risks that significantly influence tourist choice."

However, what exactly do we mean by risk to physical health? The answer to this question is not straightforward, because "perceived risk in tourism is generated by the personality traits and psychological profile of the tourist, the perceived characteristics of the tourist destination and the subjective situation of the choice of the tourist destination" (Yousfi Bachir and Schaaper 2017).

A first factor of risk perception is the feeling of security or insecurity, notably conveyed by the media. Information about violent situations (conflicts and national or international tensions) or localized epidemics can make tourists apprehensive and possibly question their choice of destination. Feedback from experiences now being widely shared through social networks is also a factor influencing the perception of risk. Criticism about hygiene or stories from sick people following their stay can have a strong impact on a tourism infrastructure. Conversely, the fact that an operator provides guarantees or even insurance is likely to reassure customers.

However, tourists' understanding of the health risk and how this translates into individual behaviors remains a subject that has been little studied to date, apart from its impact on the choices made prior to the tourist stay (destination, operators and so on). It is striking to note how many tourists are totally unaware of the risks they might incur and, even worse, how uninformed they are about seeking care at their holiday destination, relying entirely on the travel insurance and repatriation assistance they have taken out (without knowing much about the details of their cover). This is even more true for tourists coming from countries where they benefit from a strong social protection which makes them ignore the real costs of a hospitalization, for example. However, a low-cost stay can quickly become unaffordable if the tourist has to face unexpected health expenses not covered by their insurance. By way of example, Figure 2.21 shows the comparative costs of healthcare services in different countries. In France, for example, one day of hospitalization costs an average of €1,400 in a medical ward, €1,700 in a surgical ward, and more than €3,000 in intensive care. These costs vary greatly from country to country and according to the nature of the care required. On its website[35], the insurance broker ACS gives some examples of settlements they have had to pay for tourists in Southeast Asia:

– four days of hospitalization for tibial plateau fracture: US$12,300;

– seven days of hospitalization for an Achilles tendon repair following an accident: US$10,400;

– six days of hospitalization for high fever, following suspicion of dengue: US$3,000;

– two days of hospitalization for gastroenteritis: US$1,000;

– motorcycle accident with multiple fractures: US$150,000.

Tourists, who are very poorly informed on this subject and often reluctant to obtain information prior to a trip, expose themselves to the risk of poor care, which can have dramatic consequences on their health. This lack of anticipation can be explained very simply by the state of mind that prevails before a vacation departure and which was summed up by one septuagenarian French tourist we met in Senegal. She had difficulties with walking and respiratory insufficiency due to her age, but which, for her, was not a reason to give up traveling. However, she had not inquired about whether or not a doctor would be available near her vacation residence, or about hospitals or clinics in the region, and even less about the availability or otherwise of ambulances equipped with operational first aid equipment (it is not uncommon in western Africa for ambulances to be "bare" vehicles without even

35 www.acs-ami.com/fr/blog/guide-assurance/soins-medicaux-a-l-etranger/, accessed 05/18/2020.

oxygen for patients in respiratory distress). For this lady, the fact that she had taken out repatriation insurance totally guaranteed her safety.

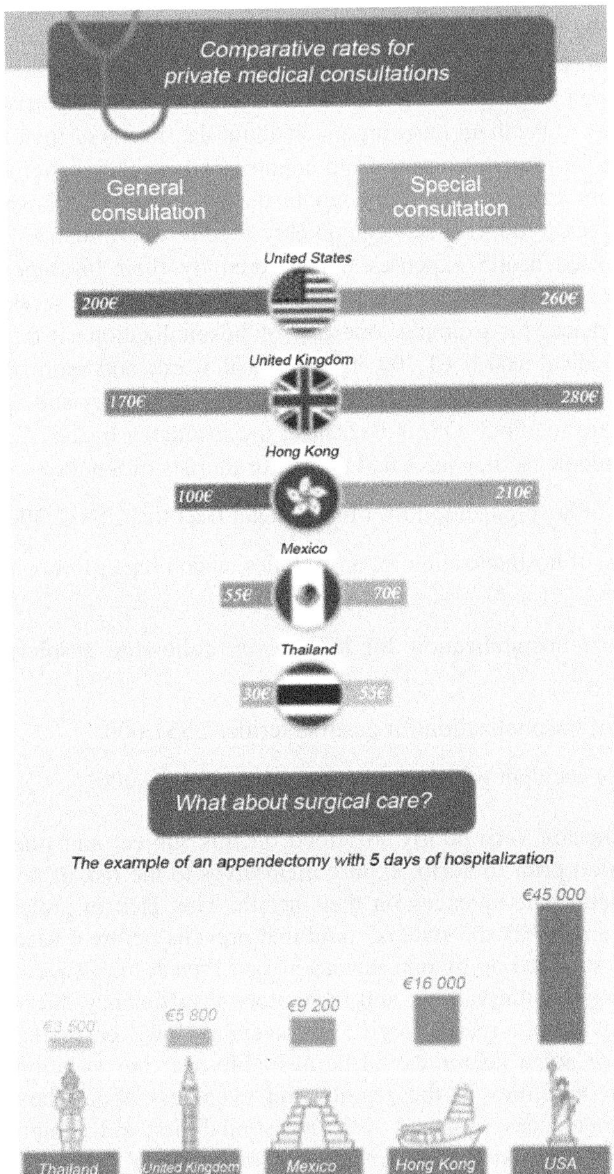

Figure 2.21. *Variations in medical and surgical costs by country (source: https://fr.april-international.com/fr, 2020)*

2.4.2.2. *Assistance and repatriation, a familiar subject but little known by the general public*

What does travel insurance cover in terms of health? What are the conditions for medical repatriation? Is it a panacea? How does such an operation work? And at what cost? So many questions that tourists are usually at a loss to answer.

According to the website of one travel insurance group,

> Travel insurance will not help you immediately in case of an emergency, and it is more important to contact local emergency services than your insurer in such cases. Nevertheless, your insurance helpline, which can be reached at any time, can help you find the nearest doctor and organize your hospitalization, and even your repatriation if your condition requires it. In addition, travel insurance will cover your care, wherever you are in the world, which allows you to leave with peace of mind.

There are two types of medical repatriation: emergency repatriation, where the local technical facilities do not allow for satisfactory treatment, and less urgent repatriation, where the patient is stabilized after initial care on site. In both cases, logistical, administrative and medical constraints are imposed on the operation. Repatriation is said to be medicalized when the presence of a nurse or a doctor is necessary to accompany the patient during the journey. The arrangements made depend on each situation and its degree of seriousness. This can range from booking simple airplane seats on a regular route to chartering a medical plane for the most urgent cases, such as an unstabilized stroke or a road accident. However, even the first case can prove extremely costly because the patient, depending on their state of health, can fly either in business class in a semi-recumbent position or on a stretcher in economy class. Two or three rows of two seats must be mobilized in the aircraft to accommodate a stretcher, plus one or two for the accompanying medical personnel, which translates into having to purchase the equivalent of six to eight seats. The patient can also travel in a specific space provided on some scheduled flights and called a patient transport compartment or PTC. The technical equipment and medications available in this specialized space are similar to those in emergency vehicles (ambulances) and enable patients to be transported under artificial respiration, to be monitored, connected to a drip and so on, and thus enables the air transfer of intensive care patients.

Health repatriation is bed-to-bed, from the place of hospitalization (including residential hospitalization in a hotel) to a hospital bed near or at home, and requires coordination between the departure and arrival medical teams. Costs therefore include ground and air transportation (airplane and/or helicopter) and personnel to provide care at each stage of the journey. These costs are covered so long as the traveler has taken out insurance when booking their trip, or via their credit card if travel insurance is included. For domestic tourism, rules vary according to national social security policies. The European Convention on Social and Medical Assistance commits the 47 signatory countries to provide the assistance provided by the legislation in force in their country to nationals of other countries who are legally resident and lack sufficient resources. In the rest of the world, in the absence of insurance, travelers requiring medical evacuation may be assisted by their consulate.

The website www.assurancevoyage.fr gives some examples of costs: "Repatriation is quite expensive since, in most cases, departure is rushed and requires the acquisition of available tickets which are often business or first class tickets. In addition to the cost of the plane ticket, you will also have to pay for the cost of your companions and the necessary medical equipment. The cost increases further if you have to take a special medical plane. In this case, the average cost is €40,000. For the repatriation of a corpse, the purchase of a coffin and the cost of transporting the body vary, on average, between €1,000 and €5,000."

French Polynesia is composed of 118 islands, 76 of which are inhabited (divided into five archipelagos) and populated by 277,700 inhabitants (2018). Ensuring the health of this widely dispersed population raises complex questions: should facilities be provided across the territory, at the risk of significant additional costs and under-utilization in the least densely populated areas? Do we need mobile doctors or, on the contrary, do we need to move the population towards healthcare institutions? The choice was made to set up a health map that "reflects the insular and demographic hierarchies of the territory" (Vigneron 1999). In this system, primary care is located in the vicinity, but secondary and tertiary care call on EVASAN (*Evacuations Sanitaires*) by air, to compensate for the slowness of maritime travel (35,000 were carried out in 1998 – source: Tntv). There are two types of EVASAN: emergency and scheduled, and both are covered by the CPS (*Caisse de Prévoyance Sociale*, Social Security Fund) for Polynesian nationals. This healthcare model can benefit the approximately 200,000 annual tourists as illustrated, for example, by a France Info report dated June 8, 2018, which relates that a 57-year-old tourist taken ill was "Evasaned" to Atunoa in the Marquesas Islands. Nevertheless, the 2015–2020 Polynesia Tourism Development Strategic Plan is completely silent on the issue of healthcare – only the absence of dangerous diseases is presented as a factor that might convince the tourist to choose this destination.

Box 2.3. *The medical evacuations (EVASAN) system: the case of French Polynesia*

3

Medical Tourism, Health Mobilities and Global Processes

When the relationship between tourism and health is mentioned, it almost always refers to the phenomenon of medical tourism. Of course, this is important, but other approaches must be considered in a broader vision that can be called "health tourism" and which includes tourism adapted to situations of disability, age, the specificities of certain categories of travelers, and so on. Finally, we must also consider that, when tourists travel, so do goods, substances (particularly pharmaceutical) and knowledge.

3.1. Medical tourism, definition(s) and trends

A study conducted in 2015 for Visa and Oxford Economics estimated that medical tourism involves about 16 million tourists per year and generates more than €56 billion in sales. Nevertheless, Connell (2006) in a text entitled *Sea, sun, sand… and surgery* warns that estimates of medical tourist flows vary enormously, partly because these tourists are very difficult to quantify (should we count individual patients or their accompanying family, at what point are they patients abroad, and at what point are they tourists?) and partly because tourism statistics do not include them as a separate category.

For a color version of all the figures in this chapter, see www.iste.co.uk/fleuret/tourism.zip.

3.1.1. *Definition(s)*

Medical tourism is defined as travel to a third country in order to seek care because it is either too expensive, unavailable or inaccessible in the country of origin. Geographer Chasles (2011) underlines

> the inappropriateness of the expression 'medical tourism', since it is primarily based on medical logic and not on tourism in the primary sense of the term. Indeed, the objective of this mobility is, above all, to improve health, not to have fun. Moreover, when the care received is major and the postoperative period is delicate, patients are unable to engage in tourism.

Furthermore, medical tourism does not include sub-national mobility, yet it is common to observe travel motivated by therapeutic recourse within a country's borders, to a referral center (in France, an example would be travel from the provinces towards Paris) or from one state to another within a federal framework, as in the United States. Nevertheless, the term medical tourism has become part of everyday language and has come to designate a set of international mobilities associated with care with a wide variety of medical activities that can be divided into two types. The first refers to comfort care (such as cosmetic surgery) and combines the health and hotel industries. The second consists of more essential, even vital, curative treatments and requires efficient technical platforms. While here, too, the health industry can be combined with the hotel industry in the form of medical tourism clusters (see below), it is also common for healthcare establishments to seek to develop and manage a complete offer.

Several factors have contributed to the development of medical tourism:

– The neoliberal turn in health policies has led to privatization of care, a lower level of reimbursement and an increase in costs in western countries (see Table 3.1), whereas it remains cheap in poorer countries, giving them a competitive advantage on the international healthcare market. This is reinforced by the fact that countries that aim to develop medical tourism have been able to raise their care quality standards, as we will see later.

– Continuing on from the neoliberal turn, and within the framework of so-called supply restructuring policies, certain industrialized countries have reduced their hospital capacities in order to reduce their healthcare expenditure, resulting in under-capacity and waiting lists that can reach several months. This is the case in the United States, Canada and the United Kingdom, as well as more recently in France, for certain specialties such as ophthalmic surgery. It can then be tempting for an individual to jump the waiting list by going abroad for treatment.

– Geopolitical and socio-economic factors are also at work. The economic crisis known as the "Asian market crisis" in 1997–1998 had an indirect effect: countries such as Thailand and Singapore found themselves with a large proportion of their population in economic difficulty and no longer able to pay full price for their health. Hospitals then saw medical tourism as a way to diversify their activities and sources of income. These countries then deliberately developed strategies focused on this niche tourism. Shortly afterwards, the September 11, 2001 attacks and the ensuing tensions diverted the attention of a section of the wealthy Middle Eastern clientele, who had been practicing medical tourism in America. Southeast Asia has benefited from these events to develop its own medical tourism, which has inspired other geographical areas, such as Latin America.

– The air transport sector has also evolved with the arrival on the market of low-cost flights that further reduce the cost of care abroad.

– Medical tourism service providers are now highly visible online, and the Internet allows the patient tourist to obtain information, compare offers and consult opinions and feedback online. In a study conducted using the example of Tunisia, Hallem and Barth (2011) identify three functions of the Internet for the patient-tourist:

> the Internet is thus perceived as a privileged source of information, allowing information to be obtained at a derisory cost. [...] It also represents a place of sociality, insofar as it facilitates, via online discussion forums, the meeting of patient tourists who are seeking to share their experiences, as well as a mutual moral support. Finally, the Internet is an effective means of establishing contact between the patient tourist and service providers, and in particular surgeons, who can thus carry out pre- and postoperative diagnoses remotely.

According to the authors' recommendation, all of this would nevertheless require public health and tourism services to take up the challenge and exercise a certain amount of control, and would require them to guarantee the security of the information posted online. Another effect of the Internet, highlighted by Eades (2015), is the packaging of medical tourism as a unique product: it is no longer necessary to search separately for a flight, hotel, clinic, cab, and so on. All-inclusive offers are now available and are very attractive.

At this point, it seems useful and pertinent to distinguish between medical tourism for care chosen at a lower cost from another phenomenon that we will call "delocalized care"[1], to which tourism is in some way subject. An example of this

1 As early as 2008, Hoerner was evoking the concept of healthcare delocalization in the book entitled *Géopolitique du Tourisme*.

second case can be American patients that are forced to travel to India for surgery due to lack of insurance, or to Mexico for certain types of care that have been relocated there to allow private insurers to make substantial savings.

Intervention	United States	India	Thailand	Mexico	Singapore
Coronary bypass surgery	113,000	10,000	13,000	3,250	20,000
Hip prosthesis	47,000	9,000	12,000	17,300	11,000
Adjustable gastric band	35,000	11,000	15,000	8,000	20,000
Rhinoplasty	4,500	2,000	2,500	3,200	4,375
Breast implants	6,000	2,200	2,600	2,500	8,000
Dental implants	1,188	1,100	1,429	950	1,500

Table 3.1. *Comparison of the cost of medical treatment in selected countries (in dollars) (source: Uchida in (Cooper et al. 2015))*

An example reported in the *New York Times on* August 9, 2019[2], is the most perfect illustration of these forms of offshore health care relevant to medical tourism.

Donna Ferguson, 56, had a condition that required a knee replacement. Although she had medical coverage through her husband's employer, Ashley Furniture Company, the cost of the surgery was exorbitant. She therefore accepted an option offered by her insurance company: to be operated on in Cancún, all expenses paid, together with a check for $5,000 as compensation for this relocation. The procedure was well established: the pre-operative consultations took place in the United States with an American surgeon. Once this surgeon was sure that the operation could be performed without any problems, they flew with their patient, who was then operated on at the Galenia Hospital in Cancún by a local surgeon. The American doctor was not permitted to perform the surgery in Mexico, but they were present in the operating room as a supervisor, which reassured their patient. Once the operation was completed, the surgeon flew back to the United States, without passing by the beach. They were in Cancún for less than 24 hours and received $2,700 (three times what Medicare[3]

2 See: https://www.nytimes.com/2019/08/09/business/medical-tourism-mexico.html.
3 Health insurance in the United States.

would have paid them). The patient continued her recovery at the Sheraton Four Points Hotel, an immediate extension of the Galenia Hospital (see Figure 3.1), and returned to the United States 10 days later (having received follow-up care and functional rehabilitation in Cancún), where she would be able to receive postoperative care in a domestic setting.

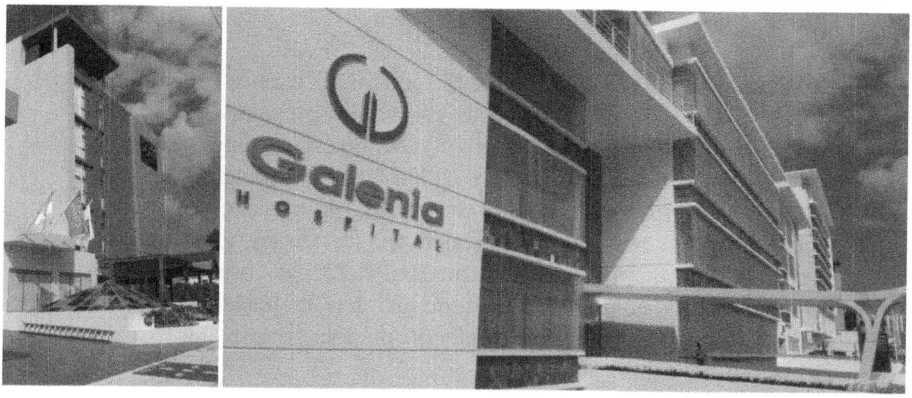

Figure 3.1. *Galenia Hospital and the Sheraton Four Points in Cancún (photos: S. Fleuret 2016)*

Several characteristics distinguish this practice from "classic" medical tourism, which is usually an individual practice: a patient in need of care that is unavailable or is too expensive approaches a medical tourism operator to find a lower-cost care provider abroad. In the example presented above, the practice was, to an extent, institutionalized as part of the health insurance package taken out by Donna Ferguson, and it is this insurance that offered the option of a delocalized operation via a joint venture between the North American Specialty Hospital in the United States and the Galenia Hospital in Mexico, which had quality standards equivalent to those of the northern hospitals and was certified by an American organization, The Joint Commission.

Even with a $5,000 check as an incentive to the patient, the insurer wins. A few figures illustrate the savings: the average knee replacement surgery costs $30,000 in the US, compared with $12,000 at Galenia Hospital; the price of a night in the hospital is approximately $2,000 in the United States compared with $300 at Galenia; the prosthesis itself costs $8,000 in the United States and only $3,500 in Mexico. In addition, the costs of the qualified personnel and all the supplies and services associated with treatment are lower… According to our calculations, we estimate that the insurer has saved around $39,000 on the cost of a similar operation in the United States.

3.1.2. *Trends and issues*

Medical tourism is part of the long history linking tourism and health, but this term only emerged at the end of the 20th century, during the 1980s, and is distinguished by the explicit use of medical treatments or operations where, in older practices (such as spas), the health benefits were indirect and not necessarily, with a few exceptions, linked to medical treatment.

> Until recently, "medical tourism" consisted mainly of wellness mobility. The care consumed was essentially preventive or curative care, but mostly concerned relatively benign morbidities. Since the 1980s, what has been incorrectly called "medical tourism" has been oriented towards diversified care and now concerns serious pathologies that require sophisticated and extremely technical care. While, at first, the most affected medical field was cosmetic surgery, for some years now, "medical tourism" has included all types of illnesses, ranging from heart defects to organ transplants (Chasles 2011).

Gradually, the terms medical tourism, health tourism and medical travel have become intertwined (Connell 2013), and together they cover very diverse realities. Although the media often focuses on examples of long-distance travel for surgical procedures, a large proportion of travel in the name of medical tourism is short- or medium-distance cross-border displacement. An exhaustive survey of medical tourism would require its own complete book (which, by the way, has already been published; see, for example, Cooper et al. (2015)), so in the following pages we will limit ourselves to outlining a few major trends (from cosmetic surgery to "reproductive tourism") and identifying the main flows and destinations, challenging the now archaic vision of the North–South divide in medical tourism.

3.1.2.1. *In the beginning was plastic surgery*

In a summer 2019 issue, the *Annales de Chirurgie Plastique Esthétique* reported on a study which ranked the main reasons for recourse to medical tourism in order of importance. Coming in at the top positions were: cosmetic surgery, bariatric surgery (to combat obesity), infertility treatment and dental care. Until the early 2000s, there were a few scientific publications on the subject of medical tourism and many still referred to health tourism inherited from the phenomenon of cure and water therapy. It seems that it is through expensive (and sometimes a bit shameful) cosmetic surgery operations in the west, that the phenomenon has developed. Breast implants, rhinoplasty, hair implants and other aesthetic procedures began to be sought after by a certain clientele outside national borders in search of the best price, since these operations were not covered by health insurance. In the United Kingdom, for example, certain orthodontic treatments considered cosmetic were not reimbursed and thus a demand was created for these treatments in low-cost destinations (Connell 2006). Initial offers appeared, such as the “scalpel safari” in South Africa (reported by Chasles (2011) and Menvielle and Menvielle (2013) among others). The Surgeon and Safari agency is the most often cited in this field, although its website no longer displays a leisure-safari offer in addition to medical services, transport and accommodation. The principle of the scalpel safari is to combine a tourist stay in a luxury hotel with a safari and a cosmetic procedure (most often a facelift). Chasles (2011) reported:

> Although sometimes the safari takes place before the surgery, most often it takes place after a few days of postoperative rest. Several types of safaris are offered, depending on the medical profile of the patients and the extent of the care received. It must be said that a safari of several days in an all-terrain vehicle can be dangerous after certain operations. Other formulas are therefore proposed, such as one-day safaris, safaris aboard authentic steam trains, or even stays in luxury residences in the middle of large national parks [...]. The average cost of this type of service is €10,000, which is the same as the price of the intervention in the United States or the United Kingdom.

This model has been duplicated in other parts of the world: Connell (2006) cited the example of the Antigua Smiles agency that promised to combine the pleasures of discovering the Caribbean with a cosmetic dental procedure.

3.1.2.2. *Recent developments*

While “in the Maghreb countries, cosmetic surgery is the backbone of the medical tourism offer to attract a European clientele, wealthy, young... and female, in India, given the more risky operations offered, it is more the professionalism and expertise of the surgeons that are advanced” (Menvielle et al. 2010). Initially, a niche market aimed at a wealthy clientele, medical tourism is now becoming more “democratic” and broadening the range of products offered. Thus, increasing numbers of essential treatments are being added to the comfort care of the Maghreb countries: for example, orthopedic surgery (such as hip and knee prostheses), chemotherapy, transplants or more recently, cures for addictions (drugs, alcohol) (Lohore 2018). “According to Mondial Assistance, the trend is more profound, which could result in a ‘demand for choice of the best care internationally’, essentially for three pathologies that are the most popular for travel today: cardiology, cancerology and ophthalmology” (Le Borgne 2007). Pharmaceutical medical tourism also seems to be progressing (Segal 2008), and this subject is developed in section 3.5 of this chapter.

Other medical fields also fall under the category of health tourism, although here the tourism dimension is debatable. These are operations that are forbidden or strongly regulated in some countries and liberalized in others. We can cite several examples here. Bariatric surgery, for instance, is reserved for adults in several countries, including Great Britain, who believe that the stomach capacity of people under 18 should not be limited. It can therefore be tempting for parents of obese children to travel to medical tourism destinations where "the customer is king" (Connell 2006).

Even more problematic, since it raises ethical, moral and societal issues, is reproductive tourism and, conversely, voluntary termination of pregnancy (VTP). Chasles and Girer (2016) studied the case of surrogate motherhood in India and noted that

> reproductive tourism is, in almost all cases, illicit, insofar as its main purpose is to circumvent a prohibition (legal or religious) of the country that we are a national of or live in: its aim is to obtain what the national law prohibits [...] it necessarily leads to travel abroad and a flow of requests to more permissive countries [...]. While reproductive tourism attracts westerners, there are also many tourists from Sri Lanka, Pakistan, Bangladesh, Thailand and even Singapore. In total, some sources estimate the number of foreigners who come to India each year for this practice at nearly 12,000. Among them, members of the Indian diaspora are particularly numerous.

The situation is complex and problematic insofar as there is no general consensus on the subject. Some countries, including France, have prohibited surrogate motherhood, others (such as India and the United States) authorize and regulate it, and others are in an intermediate position where the practice is not prohibited but neither is it regulated. However, there is more at stake than the simple medical practice of insemination followed by pregnancy: the child to be born must have rights and a recognized filiation. In France, for example, the European Court of Human Rights (ECHR) has considered that filiation should be recognized for the "mother of intention", that is, the mother who wants and raises the child, not the one who carries it; and this despite the fact that surrogacy is prohibited. This decision fills a legal void for people who have resorted to "reproductive tourism", but this decision does not impose the transcription of birth certificates, an indispensable document for which the parents of children born to surrogacy have only one recourse: adoption.

Without elaborating on it here, it should be noted that this question, like that of voluntary termination of pregnancy, or even that of the donation of certain organs, which is not always well supervised and sometimes involves a financial transaction (which generates reprehensible trafficking), raises important ethical questions and is very far from the recreational definition of tourism, even if the word continues to be improperly used to designate these practices. According to the group of non-governmental organizations, united under the banner of *transforming tourism* (see http://www.transforming-tourism.org/), the goals include "equity, justice and respect for human dignity". In the same vein, Whittaker and Leng (2016) propose speaking in terms of "flexible bio-citizenship", following on from "flexible citizenship", referring to transnational mobilities designed to accumulate "bio-value". Their argument is that for people who travel abroad for treatment (for economic reasons, or to circumvent a legal, cultural or religious barrier, or discrimination of any kind), the physical and economic ability to travel and cross borders constitutes a form of flexible social capital that enables them to access levels of care to which they would not otherwise have access. The medical tourism mobility of these people enables them to acquire "bio-value", and also modifies their relationship with citizenship and their conception of it: it is no longer strictly national, but is composed through the use of care in an international dimension. The question of inequality remains crucial, however, insofar as only a privileged fringe of the population has access to this flexible citizenship.

3.1.2.3. *Destination specialization and clustering*

> Like the globalization of trade in many sectors, the health sector is organized around a logic of specialization by country [...]. These geographic specializations allow us to see the emergence of a new world order in which specific product-market pairs are sometimes created. For example, some Eastern European countries (CEEC: Central and Eastern European Countries), such as Hungary, the Czech Republic and Romania, specialize in dental surgery and attract a Western European clientele, particularly Germans, who hop across the border for treatment (Menvielle et al. 2010).

With regard to Southeast Asia, Bochaton (2011) proposes a less tourist-centric reading (since his work refers to primary care and not exceptional or comfort treatments), but which takes into account the changes brought about by health mobility: the construction of a cross-border health basin.

> While Thais cross the border for tourism or to invest in trade, Laotians travel to Thailand for reasons more related to necessity, such as, for example, studying, searching for work, or health care. The recourse to cross-border care therefore follows from a kind of rebalancing in the face of the initial disparity that exists between the two countries [...]. Laotian patients in search of quality care and treated in neighboring hospitals weave a network of cross-border routes that give the Lao-Thai space a reticular dimension. At the same time, the actors in

> Thai private hospitals, eager to make a deeper impression on the Laotian populations living near the border, contribute to reinforcing their tailoring function and promote this networked operation within the cross-border space.

Generally speaking, it is possible to identify those countries that are resolutely targeting the medical tourism market. In the absence of reliable and exhaustive statistics, a review of the examples given in the literature on the subject makes it possible to identify the main destinations (see Figure 3.2), taking into account the bias of the predominantly English language prism of this literature, which may mask certain destinations that are less popular with North American clients, for example. In terms of major geographical areas, we can include, for Asia: Thailand (which seems to be the leader with 400,000 foreign patients per year in its hospitals), India, Malaysia, Singapore and South Korea; for the Middle East: the United Arab Emirates, Dubai, Israel, Jordan, Lebanon and Turkey; for the African continent: Tunisia and Morocco in the Maghreb and South Africa; in Europe: Spain, Belgium, Germany, Poland, Romania, Hungary and the Czech Republic; finally, in Latin America: Argentina, Mexico, Brazil, Cuba, Costa Rica and Colombia, as well as some destinations in the West Indies such as, for example, Barbados and Antigua.

Among these destinations, some, such as India, focus on generalist and low-specialization development, with a range of hospitals accredited to international standards and inexpensive access to medicines and a wide variety of practices ranging from Ayurvedic medicine to coronary artery bypass surgery. India also benefits from a widespread use of English among the population and healthcare personnel, which facilitates the acceptance of international patient tourists.

Other countries have opted for specialization, some examples of which are detailed as follows, according to Connell (2006) and Eades (2015). Hungary is particularly attractive for dental care, as is Antigua in the Caribbean; Thailand has built a strong reputation, particularly in niche markets such as sex change operations and cosmetic surgery: the anonymity that leads to distance proving to be an asset; Cuba specializes in skin diseases; Turkey is known for hair implants; South Korea is also present in the cosmetic surgery market, but has for some time been developing an oncology offering for specific organs (stomach, liver and uterus) and liver transplantation in a process of hyper-specialization; Mexico attracts a North American clientele for orthopedic and plastic surgery in Yucatán and for a broader range of care in the northern border cities and the federal capital, Mexico City. This hyper-specialization is therefore also geographical: Dubai, for example, welcomes German doctors in order to guarantee the quality of the care provided there and attract German patient tourists, while Malaysia and Singapore are particularly attractive to European and American expatriates living in Asia.

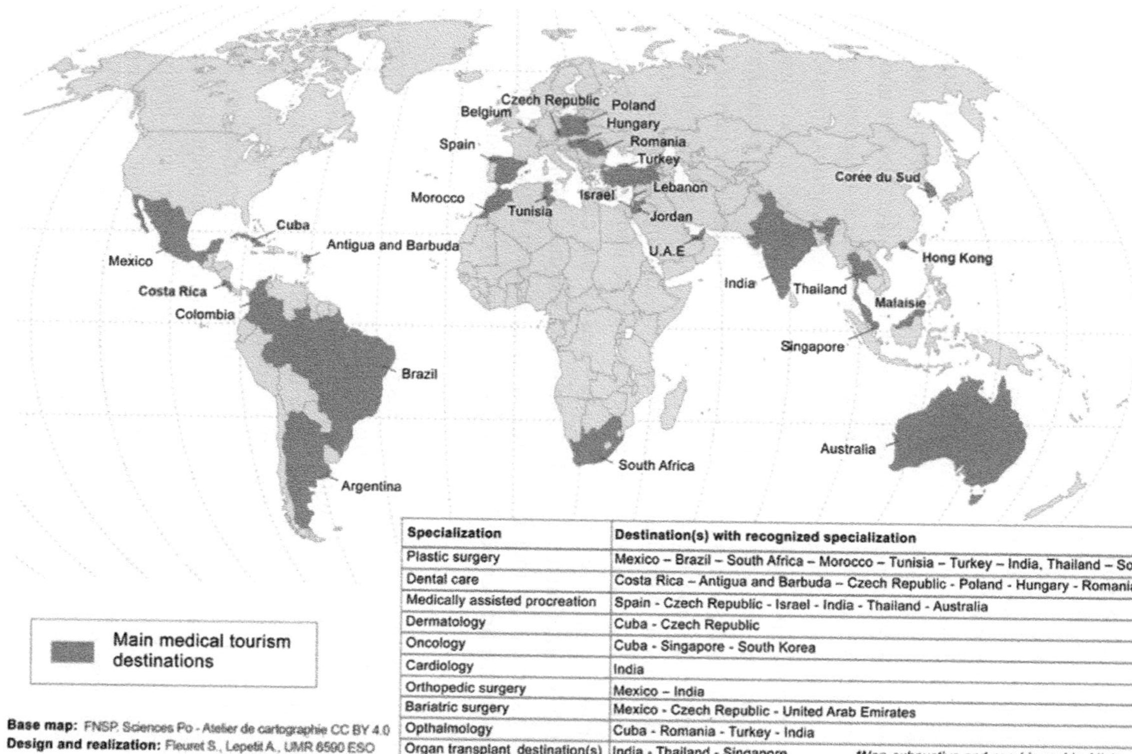

Specialization	Destination(s) with recognized specialization
Plastic surgery	Mexico – Brazil – South Africa – Morocco – Tunisia – Turkey – India, Thailand – South Koea
Dental care	Costa Rica – Antigua and Barbuda – Czech Republic - Poland - Hungary - Romania - India - Malaysia
Medically assisted procreation	Spain - Czech Republic - Israel - India - Thailand - Australia
Dermatology	Cuba - Czech Republic
Oncology	Cuba - Singapore - South Korea
Cardiology	India
Orthopedic surgery	Mexico – India
Bariatric surgery	Mexico - Czech Republic - United Arab Emirates
Opthalmology	Cuba - Romania - Turkey - India
Organ transplant destination(s)	India - Thailand - Singapore *Non-exhaustive and non-hierarchical lists

Figure 3.2. *The main destinations for medical tourism (source: literature review Fleuret S., 2021; base map: FNSP. Sciences Po - Cartography Workshop CC BY 4.0; design and production: Fleuret S., Lepetit A., UMR 6590 ESO)*

The phenomenon of geographical specialization can also be observed in initiatives such as the construction of a healthcare town on Jeju Island, Korea, where healthcare infrastructures and tourist facilities are combined and made easily accessible by relaxed legal conditions of residence for patients and their families. More broadly, a phenomenon of clusterization seems to be emerging, with or without the unity of place. Indeed, medical tourism requires several sectors of activity to be articulated: international and local transport, hotels and catering, care (surgical and postoperative) and possibly complementary leisure activities (discovery tours, for example). In order to optimize the development of this form of tourism, it is in the interest of operators in these different sectors to collaborate and coordinate themselves into clusters in order to offer complete, attractive, simple and secure packages. Connell (2006) reports the example of the Phuket Health and Travel website in Thailand, which, in addition to scheduling medical treatment, offers to take care of travel (domestic flight from Bangkok), hotel reservations, transfers from the airport to the hotel (possibility with car or taxi rental), as well as the organization of excursions, cruises or any other leisure service "for your relaxation and recuperation"! Thus, classical tourism is an integral and undeniable part of medical tourism. Nevertheless, some nuances should be noted on the subject of clustering around medical tourism. Although this is frequently highlighted in the literature, concrete and operational examples are still relatively rare and our field observations in Mexico, for example, have shown that very few of the clusters that have been mentioned actually function in a totally integrated manner. More often, they are simple and unsystematic partnerships, such as an agreement between a hospital and a hotel or local transport service, negotiated on a case-by-case basis according to patients' needs.

Finally, the geopolitical situation can also lead to calling the development of medical tourism in destinations that were nevertheless presented as market leaders into question. This is the case with Tunisia, whose tourism industry has been severely affected by the insecurity caused by the revolution in 2011 and the attacks in 2015. Tunisia enjoyed a hegemonic position in the Maghreb in terms of medical tourism, and particularly in cosmetic surgery. With a certain opportunism, Morocco, spared from political and security turmoil, has initiated an attempt to recover the medical tourism market, but without an overall strategy, the operation has only been partially successful. One example is the Marrakech Medical Center, which opened in 2015 to great fanfare in the media: it has 120 medical beds, a hotel with 40 rooms and 56 apartments. However, since its inauguration, the establishment financed by a large Emirati group has strangely been much less talked about and its success seems mixed. Tunisia has quietly and cleverly overcome the impact of insecurity on its medical tourism sector and today, seems to have flattened the curve after a decline in tourist attendance of nearly 30% around 2015, thanks to a comprehensive strategy of health tourism. This posture is illustrated by a statement by the President of the

Tunisian-British Chamber of Commerce in 2017, for whom it is now necessary "not to focus only on medical tourism, but to rethink a broader approach to health tourism that includes medical and wellness tourism, medical retirement and e-medicine"[4].

3.1.2.4. *Questioning the North–South model?*

> Medical tourism is often associated with North-South tourism, but this simplifying analysis does not reflect the reality associated with this concept. The term 'Southern countries' is imprecise and inappropriate, since some international organizations (such as the *Agence Universitaire de la Francophonie*, AUF) also include Eastern European countries under this term. We should therefore consider, in addition to North-South flows, migration flows from the North (reciprocal exchanges between Eastern and Western European countries) on the one hand, and South-North flows on the other (Menvielle et al. 2010).

For a long time, the flows of patient tourists from the South were small and consisted of the wealthiest classes in African countries, for example, seeking standards of quality or technology not available in their own countries in the healthcare systems of the former colonial powers. However, the situation has evolved: a middle class is emerging in many countries of the South (in Africa and Latin America, for example) and the demand from this social category is pulling healthcare systems upwards. The development of tourism in certain destinations (such as in the Yucatán Peninsula in Mexico or Bali in Indonesia) is stimulating investment in healthcare, and facilities for tourists are also accessible to wealthy local populations who no longer need to seek care abroad. Even more significant is the development of medical tourism in these countries, as they are also becoming receptive poles for South–South medical tourism: many patients from Persian Gulf countries go to India for treatment. At the first Africa Medical trade fair in Agadir in 2016, we could hear Morocco's desire to "capture" these patient tourists who come from sub-Saharan Africa to be treated in France and who would now find the same level of care at lower cost at the private hospital in Marrakech, for example. Nearer and cheaper… The questioning of the North–South model is therefore up in the air, but remains to be documented.

3.1.2.5. *Risks and complications*

Regularly, the media (press, TV) publish reports on the medical tourism craze. Very often, these reports follow a standardized pattern that describes a few practices (most often related to cosmetic surgery) before pointing out the risks through one or more accounts of negative experiences. In scientific literature, as Crooks et al. (2010) note, "most sources are largely speculative or anecdotal in nature, based on opinions rather than empirically observed facts". This treatment of the topic supports the idea

4 See: www.leaders.com.tn, accessed May 8, 2017.

that medical tourism carries a significant risk. Indeed, "medical tourism works when things go well. When everything goes wrong, it is a disaster" (Caccia et al. 2017). Scientific literature is full of studies on postoperative complications in patients (the majority of whom are women) operated on abroad. This is the case, for example, in an Australian study which estimated, based on the example of a knee replacement carried out in India, that the additional cost linked to a postoperative infection meant that, in the end, the operation cost nine times the price it would have cost, without complications, in Australia (Cheung and Wilson 2007). However, these studies are based on cases of people who are re-hospitalized upon return and do not count the number of people who did not experience any complications, so it is actually impossible to estimate the percentage of medical tourists who experience complications. Nevertheless, we can identify the risks and hazards and some precautions to take here.

The reported risks vary according to the nature of the intervention, the most significant work on which has been in the field of cosmetic surgery.

In a study conducted in Zurich, Switzerland, Klein et al. (2017) reviewed 109 patients (100% of cases recruited were women) for complications following medical tourism surgery, mainly for breast augmentations (39.4%), abdominoplasties[5] (11%) and breast reductions (7.3%). The main complications noted were infections (25.7%), suture dehiscence[6] (19.3%) or pain and discomfort (14.7%). These problems occur because many patient tourists underestimate both the magnitude of their operation and the importance of postoperative follow-up. Often, they only meet their surgeon a few days before the operation, who, as a result, will be insufficiently prepared. In addition, too few surgeons abroad provide follow-up care, and even fewer coordinate with a doctor in the home country. In most medical tourism destinations, the standards of the establishments and the hygiene conditions are equivalent to those found in the countries of origin and no study, to our knowledge, has demonstrated a higher complication rate abroad. Nevertheless, when a complication does occur, it reminds us that the challenge around a surgical procedure can extend far beyond the time of the operation itself, the individual surgeon's competence or the respecting of hygiene standards. It is a package that involves a team taking charge, an assessment of the risks and an acceptance of those risks by the informed patient, and then a follow-up until complete remission, which is guaranteed by western health systems, for example, but is not part of a cheap medical tourism offer. Parel-Amini et al. (2019) note that

> since the patient spends his postoperative recovery time in his "vacation" location, leisure time, such as smoking, sunbathing, hiking and other tourist activities, provides an additional risk of complications.

5 Procedure consisting of tightening the skin of the stomach.

6 Rupture of sutures or tearing of tissues.

> Long air or road trips, before or after surgery, predispose additional risks, including thromboembolic events that can be fatal. The unavailability of the surgeon, to whom the patient can turn after returning home in case of complications, can be another danger. Patients often resume contact with their surgeon from the host country by telephone or Skype. Since it is difficult to evaluate clinical status using images, the surgeon proposes monitoring and/or the introduction of an antibiotic therapy prescribed 'blindly', without prior bacteriological sampling. This causes, on the one hand, a delay in the management of these patients, who then present themselves to the emergency room several days later with an advanced infection (on average, eight days after the first signs of complications) and, on the other, a high rate of multi-resistant germs selected by the long-term antibiotic therapy.

Then, there is a risk at a different level to the medical issue, namely when a patient tourist resorts to treatment abroad because it is prohibited in their own country. From then on, ethical and legal questions will arise in case of complications once back home. Finally, according to another study, "many patients who have chosen [to undergo surgery] abroad can testify to the difficulties encountered, with numerous ultimately unsuccessful return trips often required, and resulting physical and psychological hardships that are difficult to live with and assume" (Matter 2015).

3.2. The patient tourist experience

As previously mentioned, medical tourism is a hot topic in the mainstream media, yet little is known about this phenomenon and, in particular about the patient tourist experience, beyond the few testimonies of bad experiences or complications. The patient tourist experience is split into three phases: preparing for the stay, the operation itself and the return, including part of the postoperative follow-up, since it is rare for convalescence to be totally completed during the stay. The following comments are largely inspired by an article published by Crooks et al. (2010).

Prior to the stay, the patient tourist needs information, so that they can make choices based on the offers at their disposal. They will find this information in advertising brochures, on websites or through facilitators, brokers (who negotiate rates among a group of service providers) who will act as assistants for the preparation of the trip, reservations and assistance with administrative formalities. These contacts may be located in the country of origin (Crooks et al. (2010) have identified about 20 in Canada, for example), and this proximity, as well as the fact of having an intermediary in close proximity, is likely to put the patient tourist at ease. At this stage, the main reason for deciding to have surgery abroad is principally the high cost to be borne if the operation were to take place in the country of residence (particularly for certain expensive technologies). This is related to the weaknesses and deficiencies of the medical system in force. Another motivating factor is the existence of sometimes long waiting lists in a country, which can lead to seeking faster treatment abroad. Finally, some patients will seek therapies that are not yet available in their own country, as is the case, for example, with stem cell therapies.

The choice of where to have the operation depends on several factors, the first being the reputation of the service and its quality. Language is also an important factor: it is indeed essential that patients can be treated by medical personnel who speak their native language, or a language with which they are familiar. Other factors are also considered, such as religion: it has been observed that patient tourists are more likely to seek treatment in a country where religious rites and practices are similar to their own. The tranquility and political stability of the destination and its cultural openness are also important. Finally, the "vacation" potential of the place is important for patient tourists who are inclined to look for destinations where they would spend an "ordinary" vacation. Beach, coconut palms, landscapes and climate are thus factors of symbolic attraction for medical tourism destinations, even if the patient tourist will not enjoy them during their convalescence.

Access to informed information is essential, even if there is some uncertainty due to its subjectivity. A lack of verification of information is to be noted, despite the existence of certain sites such as *Patients without Borders*, which publishes a recognized guide of resources in the field of medical tourism.

During the operation, one of the major issues, in addition to hygiene and the competence of the medical team (common to all operating theaters, whatever their location), is the way in which therapeutic choices are made. Indeed, a fundamental consideration for the patient is usually to base therapeutic choices on the criterion of least cost, which can then lead to a negative outcome.

The issue of follow-up care abroad is largely understudied, yet it is an essential consideration that goes beyond the mere hotel dimension (convalescence in a clinic or hotel). The temperatures and humidity levels in certain exotic destinations can cause discomfort and even harm the healing process. Certain tourist activities proposed may be risky (excessive physical effort, exposure to the sun, salt water, and so on).

Finally, the return home is another subject to consider because taking a plane in the postoperative phase is not a trivial matter. Certain risks are indeed increased (such as venous thromboses and pulmonary embolisms).

A final point that emerges from the literature on this topic is the psychological aspect. It is known that hospital visits are an important factor in helping patients to cope better with surgery and its aftermath. In the context of medical tourism, the patient may be away from all or part of their entourage for a considerable period of time, which may cause considerable stress and alter postoperative recovery.

Once back home, the patient returns to their national health system and usual doctor, who is not always well informed about the care the patient received abroad (especially if this care was decided by the patient alone, without consultation with their attending physician). This poses two problems: firstly, continuity of information is important in postoperative care to ensure that treatments are followed as closely and consistently as possible; secondly, in the event of complications, the physician needs to know the nature of the procedures performed and the medications administered in order to respond in the best possible way.

The patient tourist experience thus reveals the challenges around the international circulation of information in the field of medical tourism, whether upstream to guide and secure choices or downstream through access to patients' medical records.

3.3. Tourism and disability

Disability and psychological or functional incapacities constitute a field related to health with many overlaps. It is more accurate to speak of "disability situations", which occur when a person affected by an incapacity or an illness is unable to carry out daily activities. Disability can be compensated for in a variety of ways, including making places accessible. In the tourism sector, disability and incapacity situations are increasingly being taken into account, particularly in connection with the aging of a segment of the clientele, which is sometimes accompanied by a loss of autonomy that leads, for example, to difficulties in moving around, climbing stairs, and so on, which requires operators to adapt and make facilities more accessible. This subject would justify a book in its own right (which has already been written; see (Reichhart 2011)). In the following section, we will cover two specific aspects: adapted travel and its evolution, and the challenge of developing a tourist offer for the caregivers of disabled people, who very often do not allow themselves much rest.

3.3.1. *Adapted travels*

3.3.1.1. *General*

Historically, adapted tourism is a legacy of the associative movement, which has long been the pillar of social and medico-social action for the disabled. These associations offered specialized vacation stays, often apart from the medical–social establishments they managed. The associative sector also offered "travel agency"-type services, where the private for-profit sector considered the clientele unprofitable or too complex to handle. This is known as sector-based tourism (Reichhart 2011). More recently, another offer has developed for people with disabilities or loss of autonomy, this time an integrated offer, not forming a separate sector, but aiming to make the entire tourism offer accessible to all. This development corresponds to a general societal trend towards greater inclusion of people with disabilities or with disabilities that lead to loss of autonomy. The United Nations Convention on the Rights of Persons with Disabilities (2006) emphasizes the importance of promoting access to places of culture, leisure and tourist sites, and services for people with disabilities (Article 30: "Participation in cultural life, recreation, leisure and sport").

3.3.1.2. *From intentions to actions*

People with disabilities or loss of autonomy form a heterogeneous population with very varied and sometimes contradictory problems. A design that is favorable to one type of disability may be unfavorable to another. For example, a raised platform that facilitates access to transport for people with motor disabilities may represent a risk of falling for people with visual impairments if it is poorly signposted. In order to meet the needs of all, depending on the nature of the disability and the degree of autonomy/dependence, a typology approach is appropriate, based on a worldwide standard: the International Classification of Functioning, Disability and Health (ICF), which replaced the criticized International Classification of Impairment, Disabilities and Handicaps (ICIDH). The ICF identifies, classifies and characterizes disability situations according to a combination of individual factors (impairments, dysfunctions, disabilities – see Figure 3.3) and environmental factors (or situations).

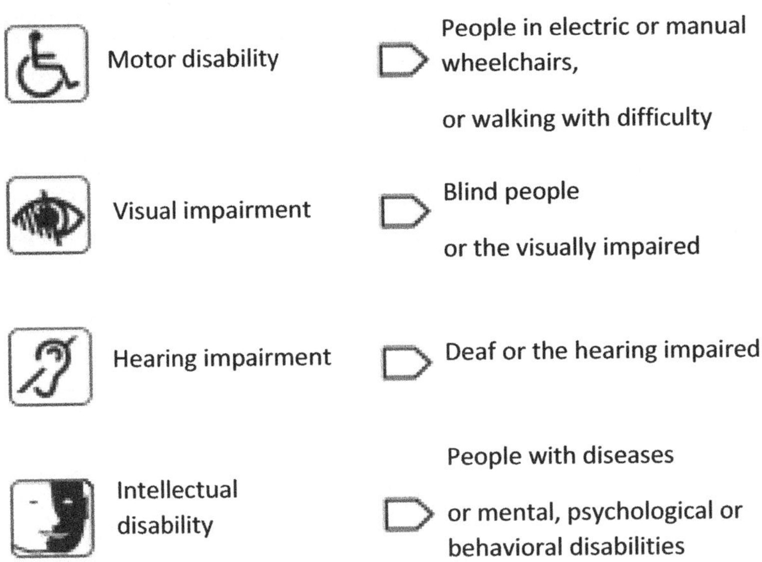

Figure 3.3. *Types of disabilities and those affected (source: Blaho-Poncé (2013))*

Compensating for a disability is achieved either by adapting the body or the environment by making it accessible. Reichhart and Lomo Myazhiom (2013) observe: "In many countries, active policies promoting accessible tourism have been put in place: often regulated by a legislative framework, which include policies for the accessibility of transport and the built environment." These policies are accompanied by labels that unfortunately "are neither standardized nor coordinated" across Europe. A multitude of initiatives have resulted in a "relatively fragmented and illegible illustration of accessibility". In France, the government has sought to remedy this by creating a "*Tourisme & Handicap*" (Tourism and Disability) label, which takes into account the four families of disabilities (auditory, mental, motor and visual) and aims to develop an adapted tourist offer integrated into the general offer. The website (see http://www.atout-france.fr/) states that "this label is the result of a collaboration between multiple actors: the ministry in charge of tourism, the professionals of the sector, the local authorities and the associations representing the disabled. Owned by the state, the accreditation was registered at the French National Institute of Intellectual Property (*Institut National de la Propriété Intellectuelle*) on February 12, 2003 as a simple collective trademark".

In spite of this homogenization approach across a territory, globally and outside national borders, non-governmental organizations, associations and groups of private sector tourism operators publish brochures and guides on accessible tourism and sometimes offer adapted tourist stays in a mix of genres that can border on conflict of interest.

Recently, one of the main online tourist reservation sites (*Booking*) added several criteria related to accessibility to its accommodation search engine. The list includes (but is not limited to) establishments that are wheelchair-accessible (ramp or elevator), have raised toilets, low sinks adapted for "persons with reduced mobility" (PRM), visual aids in Braille or tactile panels and adapted or at least level access showers.

A range of services is also being developed for people with disabilities or loss of autonomy during their stay: adapted transport from the airport or train station to the hotel, excursions, visits, rental of equipment such as a wheelchair adapted to the beach and allowing PRMs to enter the water and swim (see Figure 3.4). The aging of the western population and the associated loss of autonomy mean that this segment of tourist services is set to grow and is now a market of interest to the private sector since it is no longer limited to one population category.

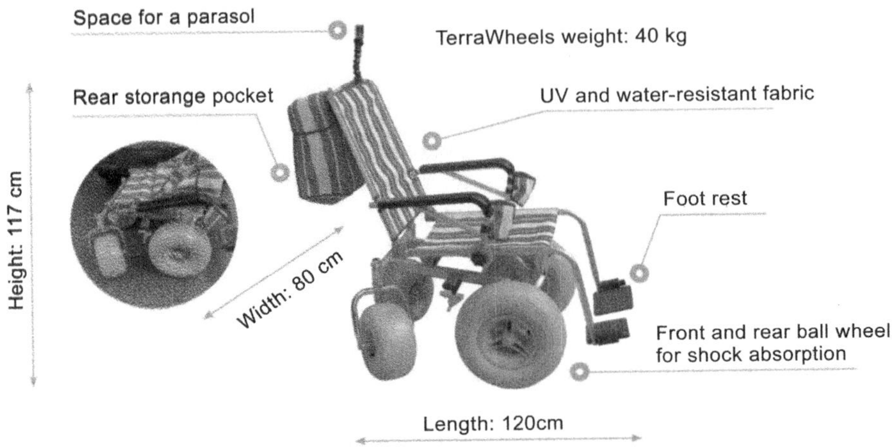

Figure 3.4. *Extract from an advertisement for the adapted wheelchair at Terrawheels beach (source: accessrec.eu)*

In tourism, as in any sector that has to adapt to disability situations, the major challenge is the continuity of travel and social inclusion, called the accessibility chain (Blaho-Poncé 2013). However, the process of seamlessly implementing accessibility is far from being completed in a majority of tourist destinations.

> It must be noted that, for the disability tourism sector, reconciling the implementation of legislative obligations for accessibility in the field of tourism and control of the quality of service provided to all users in everyday life is not yet achieved. While the preoccupation with allowing access to the attractions and services of a tourist destination is commendable, this approach is not enough to develop a tourist offer adapted to the needs of the disabled public (Blaho-Poncé 2013).

The principle of the accessibility chain is to consider tourism as a consumption chain that must be accessible at every stage and not present any breaks or discontinuities (see Box 3.1); it begins with the preparation of the trip. Information must be easily accessible and understandable (and therefore accessible to the visually or cognitively impaired, for example). At the time of departure (and later on the return journey), transport must be accessible and multimodal (such as train–plane or plane–bus connections). During the stay, the accommodation (buildings) and the places being visited, the cultural or sports activity sites, shops and places of social interaction (bars, discotheques, and so on) must also all be accessible and connected to the transport themselves.

1. How to get there.

2. How to get in.

3. How to use the infrastructure.

4. How to get out of it in case of emergency.

5. How to obtain a description of the accommodation and its adaptations.

6. How to obtain a description of possible services and their degree of accessibility (restaurants, cafés, bars, etc.).

7. How to obtain a description of the businesses and their degree of accessibility.

8. How to obtain a description of conference centers, adapted auditoriums and audio presentations of events.

9. How to obtain a description of outdoor exhibits and attractions.

10. How to obtain a description and detailed information about activities in the area.

Box 3.1. *Priorities for a coordinated policy to make a place or site accessible (source: Blaho-Poncé (2013))*

This implies an intersectoral organization, as well as an intersectoral reflection on how the destination has developed, mobilizing multiple actors: tourist offices, shopkeepers, hoteliers, leisure providers, caregivers and social workers, and so on.

There are many challenges. Very often, accessibility is only considered for each building: a hotel may have thought about its layout and made sure that it is accessible, but, for the whole trip to be adapted, the tourist must be able to get there from the train station or airport. Then, during their stay, they must be able to move around the surrounding areas, access local amenities, combine different activities, discover the culture and participate in the local social life. However, there are still too few examples where accessible tourism is considered at a destination level, which results in breaks in the accessibility chain and an alteration of the tourist experience. Faced with this situation, a promising market is developing in tourist destinations: travel facilitation. For example, the company *Go Medical* in Morocco offers tailored services to travelers with disabilities or incapacities due to age or chronic illness. The service provider will identify the needs and then propose and charge for adapted services, such as trips in an adapted vehicle, excursions with a guide and an accessible route, preparation of hotel reservations (e.g. equipping a room with an electrically adjustable bed, and so on), equipment rental and even, if necessary, "home care" at the hotel (physiotherapists, for example, or nursing care). This type of tailored service offer allows disabled people to envisage a freer form of tourism than that constrained by the brochures and offers proposed within medical–social establishments or via associations. According to Reichhart and Lomo Myazhiom (2013), a large majority of people with disabilities do not choose the place or the operator for their vacations: 70% quote an institutional prescription and 30% that of their family.

The definition of disability is complex due to the variations in the nature, origin, severity and consequences of disabilities. It is therefore difficult to accurately count the number of people with disabilities. A study conducted by "Atout France", published in 2010, provides some benchmarks for France, where 2.3 million people (approximately 3.5% of the total population) of all ages have an administrative recognition of disability. This figure rises to 5.7 million if we consider all individuals declaring a health problem or disability that limits their ability to work.

The Atout France study reveals that more than one in two disabled people declare an income of more than €1,500 per month, which makes it possible for them to consider going on vacation, regardless of the issues of autonomy and accessibility of places.

85% of those surveyed declared themselves independent on vacation, but travel was less frequent among those who needed to be accompanied.

There are variations according to the type of disability: the visually and hearing impaired go on vacation more often than the motor impaired, which can be explained by a higher level of dependence on an accompanying person.

Two-thirds of stays take place in France, with a predilection for the seaside (in 43% of cases).

As the degree of autonomy decreases, people prefer adapted commercial accommodation (such as hotels) to stays with family or friends. The Atout France study shows the relevance of the "*Tourisme & Handicap*" accreditation in making this choice, while also highlighting its limitation as a territorial network that is still too sparse. The study recommends that "adapted destinations should become more widespread, where accessibility concerns tourist sites and all environment services that are inseparable from the territory (public and social services, facilities, transport, local services)".

Seen from the point of view of the professionals benefiting from this label, the results are positive, with an impact on the loyalty of disabled clients and a positive image effect on able-bodied clients[7], despite the sometimes heavy investments required to obtain the accreditation.

For more information, see: https://www.tourisme-handicaps.org/site/assets/files/1428/etude_atout_france_21_juin_2010.pdf.

Box 3.2. *A few benchmarks for the tourism market for people with disabilities based on the "Atout France" study, 2010*

7 Nevertheless, very few professionals use this argument with their general clients.

3.3.2. *Respite tourism for caregivers*

Another segment of the tourism business that is likely to grow, although it is a niche market, is respite tourism for family caregivers. These are the parents or relatives of disabled people or people with age-related dependency (such as the spouse of an Alzheimer's patient), who devote a large part of their time to accompanying the disabled or ill person in their daily life. A study conducted in the United States estimated that this population represents approximately 54 million people, or about 16% of the US national population (Gladwell and Bedini 2004). These family caregivers (also referred to as informal caregivers) often have to balance this caregiving role with their professional and personal lives, which can become complicated. According to Holda (2015), they are the forgotten ones in health tourism, "those who care for a loved one by sacrificing their own schedule, giving up their free time for relaxation or entertainment and often even at the expense of their own health".

Whether they are assisting a person with a physical or cognitive disability, these family caregivers are very often overloaded with the tasks they have to perform and carry out in a non-professional way, that is, with a moral and emotional involvement that adds to their burden and often puts them in a situation where they become overworked or even burnt-out. Holda (2015) has drawn up a list of health problems to which family caregivers are potentially exposed as a result of the burden they carry, including: high blood pressure, stomach aches, gastroesophageal reflux, dizziness and vision problems, headaches, muscle aches, chronic fatigue and sleep problems and depression.

Moreover, this family assistance is most often provided at home, which can have a "confining" effect when the caregiver is forced to stay at home because the person being assisted is not sufficiently independent to be left alone. Leisure and tourism are rare and pose a twofold challenge for family caregivers: firstly, allowing themselves a vacation, and, secondly, being able to leave the disabled person alone to take a break. Accompanying a disabled person on vacation and going away alone are two very different things: in the first case, the family caregiver will certainly benefit from certain advantages linked to tourism, such as getting away from it all, discovering a destination and taking part in activities outside of daily life. However, the caregiver will still have to provide care, to help the person with everyday tasks, such as washing, dressing, moving and feeding.

On the other hand, traveling alone offers a real detachment from the constraints of the caregiver role, but there are several reasons why this is not so easy to implement. The first is that the emotional involvement of the caregiver often makes it difficult to leave the person they are caring for alone by entrusting them to a specialized institution or home care professionals. Psychological work may be necessary so that the caregiver can "abandon" their loved one for the duration of a vacation, or even for leisure time (respite leisure activities are also a segment of activity that should be developed, in particular as a complement to adapted trips, to offer caregivers a break for themselves). The second difficulty is the scarcity and cost of services that allow the dependent person to be taken care of while the caregiver takes a break. It is therefore necessary to consider the respite tourism offering for caregivers as a whole, a general package that includes the tourist stay and the substitution services for the caregiver during their absence. Once again, the associative sector is a driving force in this field. For example, in Indiana, United States, the Autism Resource Center, an association for parents of autistic children, has developed a pilot program to break away from non-stop caregiving. In Toronto, Canada, a respite care service offers a database of resources and services available for caregivers looking for a temporary care solution for their loved one. In New Zealand, the Ministry of Health offers a respite program that provides support (information, access to services) and financial assistance (reimbursement of costs) to allow caregivers to take time for themselves. However, there are few offers that combine substitution services with a tourist stay. One such example is that of the VRF (*Vivre le Répit en Famille*) villages in France, which are a form of respite tourism in which the caregiver's and the dependent person's vacations are articulated with separate times for each. This association was created in 2013 on the initiative of Pro-BTP (a joint social protection group serving the construction industry) and the AFM (*Association France Myopathie*). In each of the four vacation villages in France, the principle is to welcome the caregiver and the person they accompany on a daily basis at the same place. The VRF website states that by "resolving the difficulties inherent in a separation often experienced as abandonment, and by offering professional care to the person being cared for so that the caregiver can let go in complete confidence and security, the VRF concept removes the obstacles to going on vacation, which is particularly important in this type of situation"[8].

The comprehensive nature of this respite tourism offer is reflected in the role of the advisor who systematically accompanies the tourists (disabled or elderly dependents and their caregivers). This advisor is in charge of gathering the clients' expectations in order to carry out their vacation project, guaranteeing the quality of the information available to organize the stay and respite time in the best possible way, making the reservation and finally helping to put together the administrative file that will allow the aids that may be attributed to be obtained directly, for example, by the Agirc-Arrco complementary pension fund.

Although the concept may seem simple, it has come up against regulatory constraints in terms of efforts to develop and disseminate structures throughout the

8 See: https://www.vrf.fr/, accessed August 27, 2020.

country. There is no legal status for such structures which, moreover, derogate from the territorial organization of the medico-social sector, in which it is not foreseen that projects mobilize places and financing for the benefit of populations outside the territory of their location, which is one of the fundamental principles of tourism. Recently, through the law on the adaptation of society to aging (Article 45), public authorities now finally recognize establishments that offer temporary accommodation for the elderly, the disabled or the sick, while at the same time providing a vacation stay for their family caregivers.

These establishments are not subject to the criteria of compatibility of their stay projects with the objectives and needs of departmental medical and social organization plans and can therefore be established on the basis of tourist criteria in various destinations. The VRF villages are located in Anjou, Touraine, Jura and Savoy.

To our knowledge, respite tourism involving stays in separate locations for caregivers and disabled or dependent persons is not yet the subject of structured offers, and it is up to the caregivers to organize, on the one hand, their own stay and, on the other, the care of the disabled person.

3.4. Retirement tourism: from tourism to winterization

As early as the 1970s and 1980s, Cribier (1984) was studying retirement mobility, guided by a certain heliotropism and a search for living conditions more favorable to advancing age. A few years later, Clary (1991) also studied the subject and noted that this mobility was not only comprised of permanent migration, but also of "snowbirds", who flee the winter in the northern United States and Canada to settle for a few months in Florida (or more recently in Mexico or the Caribbean), benefiting from more favorable living conditions without giving up their retirement or, in the case of Canadians, for example, access to a universal healthcare system. More recently, Le Bigot (2016) has studied retired European winterers who, year after year, make a similar seasonal migration to Morocco. They are hard to identify because they statistically merge with the general tourist population, but these winterers are, according to Le Bigot, a population with heterogeneous social profiles whose motivations for undertaking these stays halfway between tourism and migration[9] are both leisure and the search for better living conditions. Nevertheless, none of these authors have extended their study of this phenomenon through the prism of health issues, even though Clary (1991) clearly identified the impacts of the

9 All of the references cited in this section mention the fact that winter migration can be a step between initial vacation visits and possible permanent settlement "in the sun" in a process that spans several years and several stays.

arrival of these "fourth age" populations on services, particularly medico-social services (see Chapter 4).

However, these long-term trips at retirement age can be linked to possible health problems associated with advancing age, ranging from a simple search for comfort (less cold and humidity for rheumatism, for example) to a real strategy of medicalized retirement tourism, based on the model of medical tourism, as illustrated by the following example (Raynal 2019). In Gammarth (Tunisia), around 20 km from the international airport of Tunis, there is a hotel residence for convalescence and retirement[10]. It is a "medical resort" (equivalent to an EHPAD (*Etablissement d'Hébergement pour Personnes Agées Dépendantes*) in France, an accommodation establishment for dependent elderly people), whose residents live there all year round, some since the establishment's opening in 2009. Alongside them, there are short-stay holidaymakers, which is what makes this establishment so unique, since it does not differ significantly from the neighboring hotel residences. Only a part of the hotel complex has been transformed into an EHPAD: certain areas such as the dining hall are shared, and families on vacation rub shoulders with the elderly without realizing that they are on the edge of medical tourism. The communication is designed accordingly, and the website clearly states that "the hotel has no stairs or steps that could hinder walking. The rooms on the garden level allow direct access to the greenery for a peaceful and secure atmosphere". "We are completely refurbishing all of the hotel rooms," says the owner. "It's up to French standards, with French comfort, at a third of the price. What we have here would cost €4,500 in France. […] If you want a house [for the elderly] with private gardens, by the sea for less than €1,500, you'll be looking for a long time and you won't find one!" says the director of the resort interviewed by Raynal (2019). Rooms adapted to the elderly or convalescent care are equipped with medical beds with anti-bedsore mattresses, a frame for orthopedic surgery, to which can be added, depending on the needs, a pulse oximeter, blood pressure monitor, oxygen, tracheal suction equipment, serum pedestals, and so on. A physiotherapy and occupational therapy room is also available. The staffing rate is about twice as high as the French average with one nurse for every 10 patients and one care assistant for every two to three patients, which is made possible by the cost of the Tunisian workforce (average salary slightly above €200 per month). Thus, despite the fact that the residents must forego French public aid, the operation is advantageous.

This type of offer, which is located on the border between health tourism and care delocalization, is still very rare and constitutes a niche market. However, it could develop as the costs and waiting lists to enter EHPADs in France and the rest of Europe are growing. The Tunisian authorities see this as an opportunity to fill the

---

10 See: http://www.resortmedical-convalescence.com/residences-hotelieres.php, accessed August 28, 2020.

hotels that remain empty during the low season. As for the owner of the resort, he is looking avidly at the potential market represented by an aging Western Europe and is considering opening a second establishment, in Turkey.

Another possible interpretation of the link between tourism and health in retirement consists, as Leroux (2010) did, of studying the moderating effect of the health variable on the behavior of seniors in their tourism activities. According to Leroux, "health is of major importance for the senior market since, as individuals age, they are generally subject to an increasing number of health-related problems, such as vision and hearing disorders, digestive problems, knee and hip problems, and cardiovascular diseases". Hoffman et al. (2017), for example, studied how North American winterers on the island of Cozumel, Mexico, adapt their drug use to the local pharmaceutical supply, at the risk, moreover, of compromising the results of the treatment initially prescribed in their country of origin.

While there is undeniably a category of poor retirees, more than three-quarters of those over 60 own their homes and have finished paying for them, which means that they have low expenses and little or no debt. Despite a drop in income when they retire, this is a category (except for elderly people who are losing their autonomy or are dependent), which has good purchasing power, time and a desire to enjoy life in a quest for well-being to which tourism contributes. In France, for example, more than five million people over the age of 60 travel every year (Leroux 2010). For this population, perhaps more than for any other, health is an important parameter. Prior to travel, it is important to take into account the higher incidence of chronic diseases in this age group (e.g. arthritis, diabetes or heart disease (Kabak 2004)), and during travel, these elderly people are sometimes more fragile in the face of the risk of accident or illness. Nevertheless, studies have shown that seniors tend to prevent this risk by having a health check-up before they travel (Neviani-Aston 2000). This act of prevention is not so common among younger people. "Getting a check-up is a guarantee of traveling well," said an elderly person interviewed by Leroux (2010). Older people also pay particular attention to their insurance: "If you have a health problem, you don't want to be stuck in the country you are visiting" (Leroux 2010).

Health can also influence the destination (e.g. avoiding high heat) or modes of transportation. For example, there is a preference for bus travel over air travel, because many older people fear the hassle of airports and the length of flights: "It takes us more than two days to recover" (Leroux 2010).

However, these precautions are limited to a health check-up, the purchase of repatriation insurance and finding summary information on the destination (quality of the facilities and food). Our own work in two destinations (Morocco and Senegal) with elderly tourists (including winter visitors) shows that the information gathered in relation to health is limited and does not include the local healthcare system. None of the people interviewed had asked about the presence of a doctor or a pharmacy that could take care of them in case of a problem, relying totally on insurance in what appears to be a relative unthinking of health in tourism. This issue is discussed in the final chapter of this book.

3.5. The backpacker phenomenon and health

We now turn to another category of travelers, much younger, the backpackers, who merit their own view through the prism of health for reasons that are quite different from the senior category.

The study of this category of travelers began in the 1970s (Ateljevic and Doorne 2004). They are referred to as "drifter tourists" (Cohen 1973) or "wanderers" (Vogt 1976), who are portrayed as a group sharing values such as the search for novelty, carelessness, a taste for risk and independence; in short, those who travel for long periods off the beaten track with a limited budget. This last point distinguishes them particularly from the young aristocratic explorers of the "grand tour", previously mentioned (see Chapter 1). They are the reflection of an era and the representatives of a form of counterculture described by Cohen (1973), having few ties, few obligations, departing from conventional standards and lifestyles, as well as renouncing the modern comforts of postindustrial society. Cohen also underlines a close link with "a drug culture", especially in Asia where the hippie movement combines drugs and spiritual travel in an itinerant experimentation, not without conflicts with the local population. However, at the time, these behaviors were not studied from a health perspective. Little by little, backpacking will develop with the increasing numbers of departing candidates, as a result of which those unbeaten tracks will become highly frequented roads, causing the phenomenon to lose its marginality. Riley (1988) described backpackers as a middle-class population, offering themselves a break in their lives, older than the backpackers of the 1970s, with a higher level of education, but not traveling like aimless vagabonds. Pearce (1990), who seems to be the author who introduced the term "backpackers" into scientific literature, adds the practice of outdoor activities (such as surfing) and the quest for healthy activities in the context of their being "beneficial for health" to this description. According to this author, the term backpackers has gradually become a marketing word for a certain type of tourist: backpacker hostels can be found in many destinations, and in France, for example, the famous Routard's Guide (*Guide du Routard*, the iconography for which is a backpacker – see Figure 3.5).

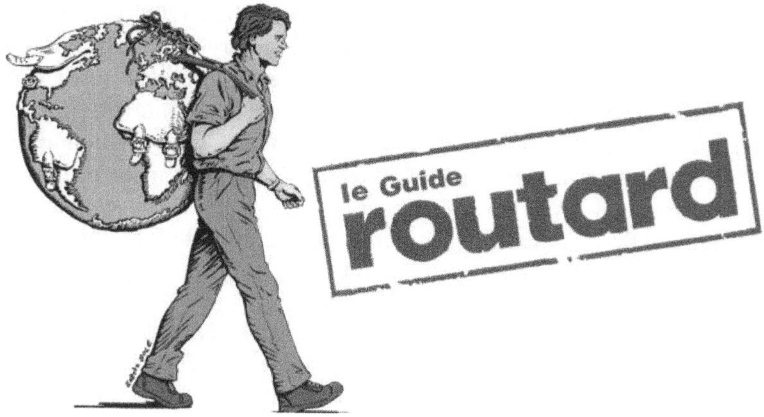

Figure 3.5. *Iconography for Routard's Guide™*

However, beyond the characterization of backpackers (which evolves as western societies change), what interests us here are the relationships of this category of tourist with health, which can be read according to two main threads: the assessment of risk (including drifts in the form of addictions) and the ways in which they use (or do not use) healthcare and alternative health practices.

3.5.1. *Risk assessment and risk taking*

Leggat and Shaw (2003) asked: Are backpackers a more risky population than other tourists? According to these authors, the backpacker could be inclined to take more risks for their health and physical integrity than people on organized trips or business tourists. The reasons for this are the young age (in general) of backpackers, their propensity to take part in adventure sports, to travel to remote destinations or underdeveloped countries, to use cheap, unsafe means of transport, to rent accommodation in unhygienic conditions, and so on. According to Richard and Wilson (2004), backpackers do what they want, their adventures and experiences make them who they are and thrill-seeking and risk-taking seem to be an integral part of backpacking. Also, because they travel cheaply, they will be less careful about food and more exposed to food-related infectious diseases (such as diarrhea). For the same financial reasons, they may face difficulties in paying for the care they need (see below). Conversely, the youthfulness of this population is a protective factor: when we are young, we are more likely to be healthy and our bodies are more resilient.

According to various studies quoted by Leggat and Shaw (2003), between 2/3 and 3/4 of backpackers have experienced an illness or injury while abroad. The most commonly reported problems are gastrointestinal infections, ear infections (often related to snorkeling), migraines, burns, musculoskeletal injuries (from falls or accidents) and various parasites contracted in unsanitary water environments. Other studies have shown that hepatitis A virus infections are much more common among backpackers compared with other categories of travelers in developing countries (Steffen et al. 2003). The disease is acquired orofecally, often through ingestion of contaminated food or water (see section 2.1.1).

Some activities are associated with specific increased risks. For example, in Australia, rafting is correlated with a higher incidence of leptospirosis (bacterial disease). Rickettsiosis (tick-borne fever) is associated with trekking in the rocky mountains of North America. Both of these examples are not risk-taking behaviors, but exposure to potentially pathogenic environments due to the places visited (white waters, forests) and the activities practiced.

Other increased risks among backpackers have been highlighted in the scientific literature, this time linked to behaviors more frequently observed in this population. Drug use is implicated in one in five cases of psychiatric problems. Non-compliance with preventive health advice is also a concern and can be observed in relation to multiple health problems: malaria, for example, requires prophylactic treatment (see Chapter 2), which is not always followed. Chatterjee (1999) observed, from a case study in India, a lower use of anti-malarial drugs among backpackers compared with other tourists visiting the country. Finally, two points merit specific attention: sexuality and the use of psychotropic products of varying degrees of illegality. A Danish study conducted at a youth hostel in Copenhagen showed that only one in five young guests had condoms with them and that only half of the men and none of the women interviewed reported using condoms during sex. Despite the bias due to the small sample size, this study is instructive and highlights the exposure of young backpackers to sexually transmitted diseases (STDs), with HIV–AIDS being the most common.

Finally, two common characteristics of backpackers may constitute risk factors that aggravate health risk factors. Firstly, they are long-distance tourists who go on long-term trips, yet this long trip duration increases the likelihood of experiencing health problems (Mansanguan et al. 2016). Secondly, the backpacker identity includes a rejection of the mainstream and the narration of an experience that is original and off the beaten track, uninfluenced by dominant ways of thinking (including medical discourse), seeing themselves as anti-tourists (Welk 2004). For example, coming close to danger, contracting an exotic disease and being cured of it are valued narrative elements. Cutting back on the accommodation budget to go scuba diving will remain in the narratives as a wonderful underwater experience and not as a time when they caught scabies.

This alternative posture, of defiance towards "the mainstream", can extend as far as a rejection of what the healthcare system represents and lead to less use of it.

3.5.2. *Seeking care and searching for alternative practices*

A study in Thailand (Mansanguan et al. 2016) of 420 backpackers of both genders (median age 26 years) examined their attitudes towards health. The study found that only 58% had visited a doctor in preparation for their trip. Only a small number had experienced a health problem during their trip (10.2%), which is much lower than what is usually described in the literature, but the problems encountered were classic, with diarrhea and stomach aches topping the list of pathologies (see above). What is interesting in this study is that it addresses attitudes towards the disease. In one-third of the cases, the person recovered without treatment. A quarter treated themselves by self-medication, either from their own medicine kit or by buying over-the-counter drugs from a pharmacy without a prescription. Only 1 in 10 backpackers who were sick went to a healthcare facility. When asked about the impact that this health problem had on their trip, 72.1% said it had no significant impact, 23.3% had to postpone a stop or an activity and only 4.7% had to give up a trip or activity altogether. Ultimately, this study shows that in a large majority of cases, the health problems encountered by backpackers are moderate and do not have a significant impact on their stay. However, in a few cases, the most serious ones, the problem can have significant consequences: the case of one Australian tourist, who we will call Sam to preserve his anonymity, speaks for itself. We met Sam in a hospital in Denpasar, Bali, where he had just had part of his right leg amputated. A few weeks earlier, he had been the victim of a scooter accident, a fall from not too great a height, but in shorts and flip-flops: the body was not protected and Sam suffered an open fracture of his ankle. Quickly admitted to the hospital, his fracture was reabsorbed and sutured but he had no idea of the cost of the hospitalization and had not taken out any insurance. When presented with the bill, he left the hospital, stating that he could not pay and continued his convalescence in a low cost hostel. Without proper care and satisfactory hygiene conditions to change his dressings, the wound became infected. Fearing the cost, Sam did not return to the hospital where he would have been prescribed appropriate antibiotic therapy and instead turned to a traditional healer recommended by another backpacker. This treatment had no effect and quickly turned into septicemia. Experiencing high fever, pain and seeing his tissues necrosing, he finally decided to go back to the hospital emergency room where his life was saved but not his leg. This story may seem anecdotal, but it is indicative of the problems posed by the health of backpackers: how can we raise awareness among this population that is defiant towards the healthcare system, distrustful of, and even rejecting, preventive measures, young and carefree, and therefore often poorly insured? How can we ensure that these singular tourists do not renounce care because of ideology or a lack of means?

Another factor adds to this risk of not seeking healthcare, namely a greater propensity among backpackers than among other tourists towards seeking alternative experiences in health-related fields. Some of these experiences involve traditional and relatively well-supervised alternative therapies (*Ayurveda, Qi Gong*, acupuncture, and so on) and do not present any real danger, so long as they are not used for pathologies that these practices cannot treat. Certain practices (such as detox, 100% vegetable diets and fasting) also may not, if supervised by a nutritionist, pose a problem. On the other hand, other alternative therapies raise more questions, and the use of marabouts and other shamans, and traditional pharmacopoeias (sometimes bordering on psychotropic drugs) can be harmful. For example, sectarian aberrations linked to neo-shamanism are reported in the Riviera Maya in Mexico (this subject is developed further on). The subject is thorny because the backpacker wishing to visit a country by immersing themselves in its habits and customs can, in all sincerity, include traditional care in this. Work remains to disentangle good and bad practices and formulate appropriate recommendations to travelers so that these experiences do not end in disaster.

3.6. Circulations, vernacular knowledge and health versus tourism and globalization

The movements of tourists, whatever the scale, are accompanied by several forms of mobility, both material and immaterial. In the relationship between tourism and health, material flows take the form of substances (such as medicines, traditional remedies and plants), which may be the very object of the trip in a tourism that is no longer medical, but pharmaceutical. Immaterial flows are forms of knowledge or beliefs to which the tourist is initiated and which they will bring back home and sometimes remobilize into their daily life, by adapting it to their way of life in a process of transnationalization. This notion, which assumes that globalization processes tend towards standardization of cultures and identities in a transnational way through mobilities, migrations and diasporas, has been applied to health and well-being practices. An example is the work of Hoyez (2008) on yoga, a traditional Indian bodily and spiritual practice that has been (in a process of knowledge circulation), "reinterpreted in the light of various theories, [...] and has developed principally in large European (American) and Indian cities, where thinkers and practitioners reside". Yoga has thus been reinterpreted by, and for, these urban populations. Thus, from traditional knowledge, we have moved to individual globalized practices that are well established in the daily lives of many Europeans

(Americans) or Indians, which refer as much to a so-called modern way of life as to a "Hindu tradition". Hoyez has thus defined transnationalization around health-related practices or knowledge as the way in which "individuals and groups are linked by networks that occupy space and places on a global scale [...]. The process of globalization of yoga then corresponds to the concordance of the sum of individual actions localized in the world space". Tourism can participate in this phenomenon, notably through discovery trips or retreats in India during which the practice of yoga (or other alternative treatments, such as ayurveda) are the main reason for the trip. In the following section, we will firstly deal with material flows from the pharmaceutical tourism angle; then, we will return to the immaterial flows of practices and knowledge from the case of shamanic tourism.

3.6.1. *Substance circulations and pharmaceutical tourism*

Segal (2008) asked the question: "*Is pharmaceutical tourism just around the corner?*" His question is based on observations similar to those described earlier in this book about medical tourism, namely the prohibitive cost of certain pharmaceutical treatments and their non-reimbursement by medical insurance companies, which encourage patients to seek cheaper treatment abroad.

Some over-the-counter medicines and others requiring a medical prescription in France are considered illegal substances (drugs) in some countries (e.g. in the Maghreb or in Southeast Asia). Therefore, they cannot be imported without prior authorization from the local Ministry of Public Health. If you go to a restricted country without this authorization, you will not be allowed to enter with the drug and you may also be prosecuted according to national laws. If these drugs are prescribed for you by your doctor, you must carry a certificate from the doctor confirming that the drug is prescribed for you. This certificate, written in English, must mention the type of pathology, the commercial name of the medication(s) concerned and the dosage. In some cases, tourism professionals are not aware of their duty to warn their clients of this risk and provisions or that these warnings are drowned in a mass of information on the general conditions of use (GCU) that nobody reads in the case of reservations booked online. The WHO publishes a nomenclature (the International Non-proprietary Names, INN), and it is quite easy to find out about the molecules to check if we are dealing with an equivalent of a known drug which may have a totally different name from one country to another. The name of the molecule remains constant, and the INN lists more than 7,000.

Pharmaceutical tourism is very directly concerned by the issues related to the legality or illegality of the circulation of certain substances. As Segal (2008) points out perfectly:

> Surgical tourism is about a one-time event, but there are diseases that require daily treatment over the long term. Most people would rather stay in their home country (the United States in Segal's example, NDA) than move to a third-world country for treatment. Right? However, what if the patient buys their treatment abroad and then returns home for care? Isn't that smuggling? Of course it is, but here the stakes are high (people's health) and the value of the drug components is sometimes much higher than the value of drugs traditionally listed as illegal. Are we really going to arrest these sick people on the grounds that they have smuggled in substances to save their lives? I doubt it.

A press article published in the French newspaper *Le Parisien*[11] corroborates these statements. It states that, despite the absence of figures,

> experts note an increase in travel to buy cheaper drugs or those that are simply not available in France, despite the risk of buying a counterfeit that may have no effect or, worse, may poison the person. This observation is made in particular through airport seizures of products imported by individuals – which is prohibited – as well as by traffickers who flood Europe with copies, not to mention purchases online, "a practice that is exploding", according to the *Académie de Médecine*.

According to *Le Parisien*, the difficulties in accessing certain new and expensive treatments are pushing "doctors to select beneficiaries and advise others to seek treatment… abroad. This is how patients go to countries like India where real – legal – specialized care channels are organized". One example speaks for itself: a drug prescribed for the treatment of hepatitis C could benefit 140,000 patients in France, but only 26,000 have access to it because the three-month treatment is billed to Social Security at €41,000 per patient (source: *Le Parisien*), whereas a generic version can be found in India for €900. The same is true for a large number of anti-cancer drugs, but, since their mode of administration is more complex, it is very difficult for a patient to go abroad to acquire and self-administer them. Nevertheless, we are seeing the development of low-cost pharmaceutical channels from countries that specialize in generic drugs in response to the "incommensurable positions taken by the pharmaceutical industry and NGOs militating for the right to health" (Vaguet 2018). This is a supply of generics in opposition to patent policy and in particular to "evergreening" (which consists of marginally changing the formula of a drug when it is about to drop into the public domain in order to extend the private exploitation patent). Among the countries that have opted for this specialization are India, as well as Bangladesh, Egypt and Morocco. China, on the other hand, feeds the market with

11 See: https://www.leparisien.fr/societe/sante-l-inquietante-croissance-du-tourisme-pharmaceutique-05-04-2016-5687935.php, accessed October 21, 2020.

counterfeits. On the side of the client countries, new forms of structures are emerging, such as central purchasing functions for imported medicines (in Australia, source: *Le Parisien*), some of whose members are charged with supply during tourist stays. Thus, a geography of parallel drug circuits is emerging (see Figure 3.6).

Other reasons for buying abroad include the use of drugs that are prohibited in France, which is the case with cannabis derivatives. For example, a drug prescribed as an adjunct to the treatment of muscle pain for patients with multiple sclerosis obtained a market authorization in 2014, but is still not yet commercially available in France, and patients are forced to go to Switzerland to buy it, at the risk of a customs check. In 2020, testing on anti-pain treatments derived from cannabis was announced in France, but the situation is evolving very slowly and patients continue, in the meantime, to practice pharmaceutical tourism.

Pharmaceutical tourism is most frequently observed over short distances, in border areas, as shown by the following three examples.

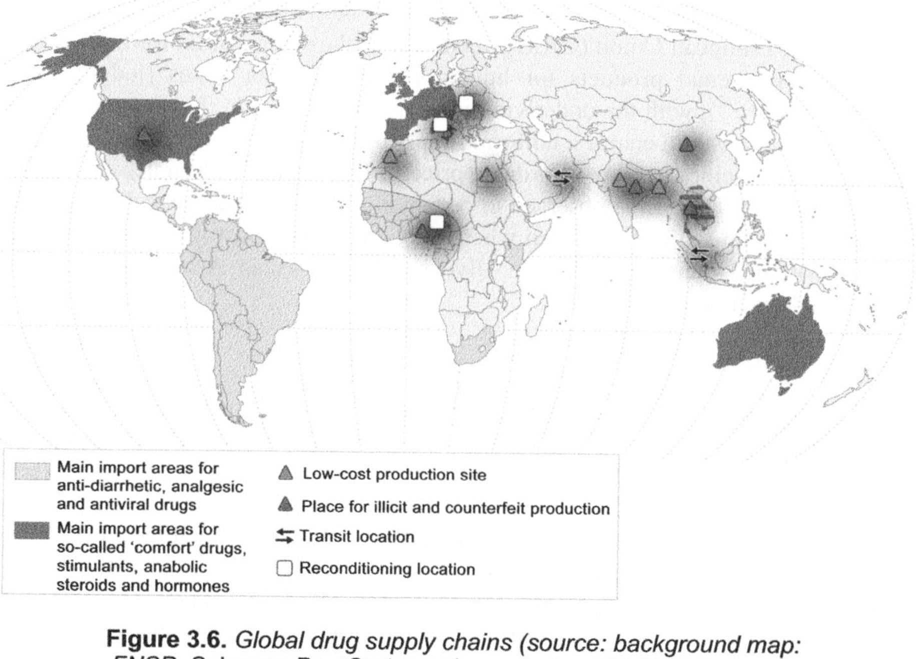

Figure 3.6. *Global drug supply chains (source: background map: FNSP. Sciences Po - Cartography workshop CC BY 4.0; design and production: Fleuret S., Lepetit A., UMR 6590 ESO)*

3.6.1.1. *Example 1*

In an article published in the newspaper *Le Monde* on April 15, 2009, J.-P. Stroobants presents the village of Ulvenhout, located near Breda, but especially close to the Belgian border and the city of Antwerp, as a village that is "clean, but probably not worthy of being in the guidebooks". However, according to the author, many tourists come from Belgium, the aim of these "walkers" being to buy medicines that are much cheaper than at home. This price difference within the European Union's free trade zone was born from the possibility of applying a model from New Zealand, the so-called "Kiwi model", in the Netherlands (and not in Belgium), which consists, within a range of drugs (such as antidepressants or painkillers), of applying a large discount to a single brand, often a drug that has reached the end of its patent life. Other brands are no longer reimbursed, which leads to a general drop in prices. Although limited, this system has created a differential on both sides of the border, provoking a reaction from the Belgian pharmacists' unions, which have raised the specter of drug tourism, or a system of parallel imports that would eventually threaten the very active pharmaceutical research in Belgium. Far from wanting to counteract these price differences between countries, the Court of Justice of the European Union (CJEU) ruled against the setting of uniform prices for the sale of medicinal products for human use by member states (judgment of October 20, 2016[12]), with the underlying ideology formulated in this judgment "that price competition would enable a uniform supply of medicinal products and access to prescription medicines at more affordable prices". This example illustrates the kind of shopping tourism that can be observed in certain border areas with very different tax policies on certain products, or even where duty-free zones exist. Thus, an Antwerp resident will buy their painkillers in Ulvenhoudt, just as an Ariegean can go to Andorra to buy cigarettes.

3.6.1.2. *Example 2*

Along the borders that Laos shares with its neighbors (Vietnam, China, Thailand, Cambodia and Myanmar) are entry points for various and diverse pharmaceutical products (Quet et al. 2018). Medicines cross borders discreetly in travelers' suitcases, or even in containers that customs authorities cannot control due to lack of tools and sufficient human resources. In December 2014, monotherapies produced in Vietnam to treat malaria, and yet banned from sale throughout the sub-region (following a 2006 WHO recommendation citing the emergence of forms of resistance), were found in the pharmacy of a large public hospital in the Lao province of Champasak. This episode highlighted the porous nature of the border between Vietnam and Laos in terms of controlling the circulation and sale of medicines and revealed the unscrupulous practices of certain manufacturers, ready to

12 See: https://www.fhf.fr/Europe-International/Les-arrets-de-la-Cour-de-justice-europeenne/libre-circulation-des-medicaments.

do anything to sell their stocks of medicines. The geography of Laos partly explains this phenomenon: the country is very stretched out and circulation is difficult. Many regions are far from the capital Vientiane and much closer to cities on the other side of the border and the services they have to offer, especially in health (Bochaton 2015). While cross-border use of hospital care (from Laos to Thailand) is well documented and often linked to another reason for travel, such as trade, business, tourism and family visits (Bochaton 2011), the circulation of medicines is less well documented. In contrast, the circulation of substances associated with diaspora tourism has been studied, for example, between Laos and the United States among the Hmong diaspora (Bochaton 2019). By diaspora tourism, we mean returning to the country of origin during vacation stays, which are an opportunity to bring back products that are sometimes unavailable in the country of expatriation. Medicinal herbs and traditional pharmacopoeia therefore form part of the products that travel in tourists' suitcases or by mail, which allow expatriates to maintain a link with their country of origin through recourse to traditional medicines and which allow caregivers who have themselves emigrated to rebuild a transnational healthcare offering in the destination country.

3.6.1.3. *Example 3*

The proximity between Mexico and the United States of America provides examples of "pharmaceutical tourism" born from the differential between the cost of drugs and the failures of the American health insurance system. In 2016, 8% of Americans reported purchasing drugs abroad (source: Slate[13]).

The border state of California in the United States has a large population of Mexican origin. This population tends to cross the border into Mexico for various purchases when the cost differential is advantageous, which is the case for drugs and various health services. For example, in Orange County, a suburb of Los Angeles, 33% of the population is Hispanic and more than a third of this minority is too poor to have health insurance. In response to this reality, *Salud con Health Net* was launched in 2000, which is the adaptation of a cross-border health maintenance organization in California. As a reminder, HMOs are insurance schemes that select a list of healthcare providers and establishments with which they sign agreements. Policyholders are required to seek care from this list if they want to receive reimbursement. Before the creation of *Salud con Health Net,* a person of Mexican origin who returned to Mexico for treatment paid less but was not reimbursed. Now, thanks to this cross-border scheme, policyholders can travel to Tijuana to see a doctor and buy medicine while still receiving their US insurance. Other insurers have similar arrangements: for example, *Blue Shield* offers a program called *Access Baja* (for Baja California, the Mexican state next to California).

13 See: http://www.slate.fr/story/187461/utah-fonctionnaires-tourisme-medical-mexique-canada.

Initially intended for the diaspora, these cross-border medical coverage programs seem to be attracting another category of medical tourists: snowbirds. Miller-Thayer (2010) studied cross-border health-related use among this population, which she defines as follows: "A snowbird is someone 55 years or older from the northern United States or Canada who spends the winter months in the warm southern United States for five or six months between October-November and the end of March." The Mexican border represents an opportunity for them in terms of healthcare: with healthcare and medications being cheaper on the Mexican side, a portion of the lower-income US population is trying to optimize their healthcare costs by making the best use of resources available on both sides of the border by staying near the border for several months. Miller-Thayer was able to observe the practices of these snowbirds at the borders: some come to spend a few months in their motor homes in the south and take the opportunity to cross the border for one or more days; some make the trip by private car, and others take advantage of organized bus tours to seek dental or eye care that they cannot afford in the United States, or to buy the medication required for several months of treatment for their chronic illnesses. These practices are also visible in urban space. Miller-Thayer counted 86 dentists, 24 pharmacies and 29 opticians in the small border town of Los Algodones, nicknamed *Molar City*, which had a population of only 5,474 in 2010.

This phenomenon of cross-border healthcare is not limited to the states close to Mexico, which is why it can be called medical or pharmaceutical tourism, because it is accompanied by a stay in the country. This can also be instituted in a system like that in Utah, separated from Mexico by Arizona, where a special insurance program was created in 2018 for government employees. The principle is the same as previously discussed for the use of surgical tourism in Cancún (see section 3.1.1): rather than reimbursing the very high US price of drugs, it is more cost-effective for the state to pay its public servants for a trip to Mexico with a $500 annual bonus. A pilot study conducted on 10 patients would have saved $225,000 in one year (source: *Slate*).

While the primary motivation for policyholders to use this pharmaceutical tourism system is access to affordable medicines, ABC News also reports the story of an employee who had enough health coverage to receive full reimbursement in the United States, but still activated the health tourism option in order to take a trip to Mexico, paid for by her insurance.

It is appropriate here to reiterate the limitations of using the term "tourism" to describe cross-border practices of seeking care or pharmacopoeia. Although travel is most often accompanied by a hotel stay and, in a large number of cases, by an experience of local discovery (visiting, eating out, and so on), the main motivation for travel remains compensation for a lack of access to healthcare in the country of origin. However, pharmaceutical tourism has another component that corresponds more to the classic tourist experience, and focuses on traditional practices and knowledge through visits during a classic tourist trip, like visiting a museum or a monument.

3.6.2. *From traditional health knowledge tourism to shamanic tourism*

In many destinations, traditional health practices and associated substances are promoted for tourism. We previously mentioned argan oil, which was promoted in southern Morocco as a traditional remedy both for its nutritional properties and as a massage oil.

We have also mentioned Asia, where massage parlors abound in tourist areas of Thailand and Bali, where they can be combined in a tourist offer with other products, such as herbal concoctions or teas with relaxing properties.

Far from being reserved for a niche clientele, these tourist offers based on age-old knowledge target mass tourism, as illustrated by the following example: the medicinal plant hut in Yodzonot, Mexico (see Figure 3.7).

Located west of Valladolid in the state of Yucatán, Yodzonot is a small village that borders the main road that connects the major archaeological site of Chichén Itzá to the coastal tourism area of Cancún. In Yodzonot, there is a cenote, a natural well eroded from the karst plateau and filled with water suitable for bathing (see Figure 3.8). This cenote is a stop for buses making day trips to Chichén Itzá from Cancún. At the exit of the bathing area, there is a hut with a sign "*medicina tradicional*" that invites tourists to enter a Mayan herbal store where a local woman, trained in herbal medicine thanks to a philanthropic program funded by the WK Kellogg Foundation, provides traditional practitioner advice on the treatment of various ailments (such as migraines, stomach aches and joint pains) and sells packets of medicinal plants that she also offers to send directly to the tourist's home by parcel post. Observing the comings and goings of tourists in this place shows that the medicinal stall is becoming a stop on the bus tour, like any other souvenir store.

The interest in traditional pharmacopoeias represents a minor segment of the tourist activity. Yodzonot welcomes 40,000 visitors per year, and only a small portion of them visit the traditional health hut (the traditional practitioner keeps a register which, for the year 2017, preceding our visit, listed 150 names).

In the example below, pharmaceutical tourism is an opportunistic activity, with herbal stores attracting classic flows whose motivation is unrelated to health or well-being.

It is different in the next example, that of shamanic tourism motivated by a quest that mixes health, well-being (even happiness) and spiritual, mystical or religious experiences.

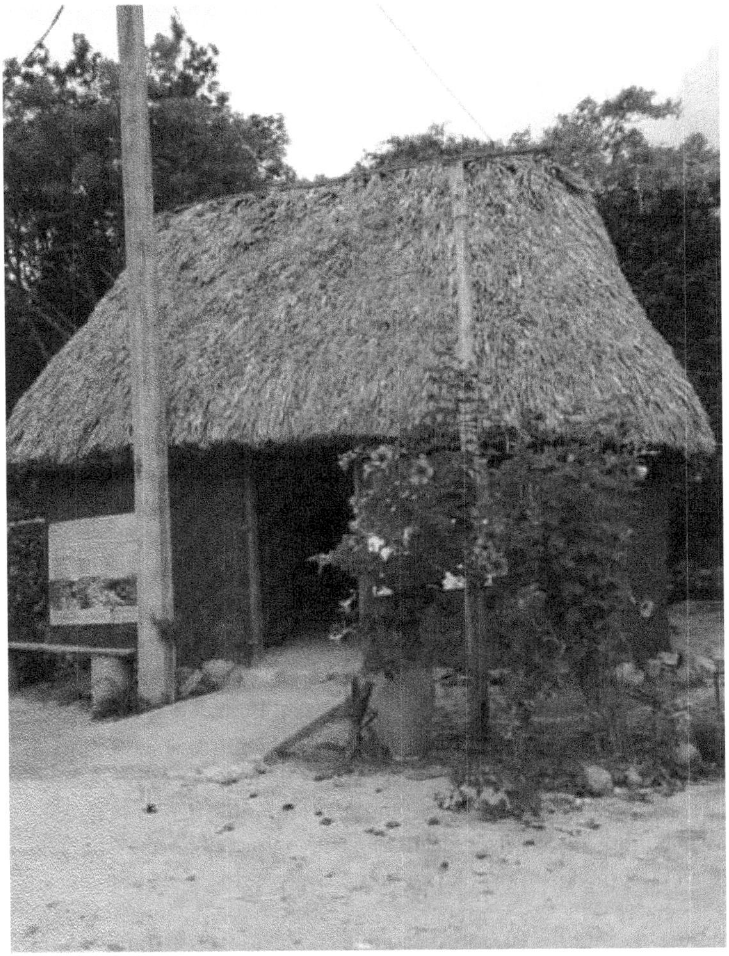

Figure 3.7. *Medicinal hut in Yodzonot (photo: Medicina Tradicional Xunáanil Ka Ax 2017)*

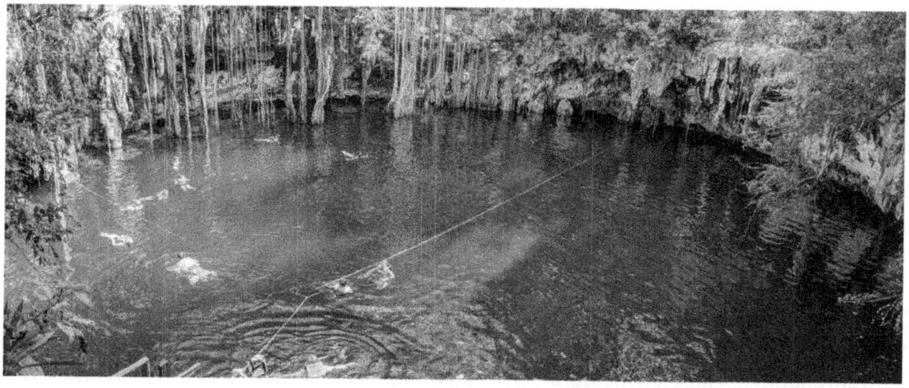

Figure 3.8. *The Yodzonot cenote in Mexico (source: www.lescovoyageurs.com)*

The Mazatec Indians in Mexico became known in the 1960s for their ritual use of hallucinogenic mushrooms and thereby aroused the interest of western tourists. It was

> following the media revelation of the "cult of sacred mushrooms" by Wasson, a New York banker with a passion for mycology [that] the chief town of the Mazatec highlands, Huautla de Jimenez, became a mecca for mystical tourism. As foreign visitors return each year during the rainy season, "magic mushrooms" season, the Mazatecs have mobilized the elements of shamanism for ethnic and cultural ends, but also for commercial and tourist instrumentalization (Demanget 2015).

As Demanget (2015) points out, the object of the tourist visit here smells of sulfur. "What is consumed are not 'commodities', but individual experiences over which hangs the specter of drugs and profane experience. These tourist practices are particularly prone to hostility for being more generally associated with tourist pleasure deemed guilty in our societies". In western societies, drugs are seen as addictive and therefore do not mix well with the idea of pleasure, and yet there are many tourists tempted by the exploration of its inner potentialities that shamanism proposes through, here, a hallucinogenic substance. The traditional character of this practice in some way legitimizes this: it is about a return to the source, to a knowledge or to secular practices. In the 1960s, this attraction for various practices related to shamanism was popularized by several artists, first of all the *Beatles*, who widely publicized their stay in an ashram in Rishikesh, India, where they discovered transcendental meditation (and consumed LSD…). After being abandoned by Maharishi Mahesh Yogi's organization, the site was taken over in 2012 and renamed "The Beatles Ashram," making it a major tourist attraction.

However, the Beatles' stay in Rishikesh did not end in idyllic fashion, but with a hasty departure against a backdrop of accusations of breach of trust. At the end of this stay, George Harrison and John Lennon would display positions related to the New Age movement, a syncretic trend of multiple practices and heterogeneous beliefs. After a decline during the 1980s and 1990s, the New Age movement is now experiencing a resurgence in interest. While the first wave of this movement was quite clearly linked to India and led the first backpackers to make "initiatory" trips, the new wave seems to be more geographically diffused and we find experiential, neo-shamanic tourism in many destinations. In the Amazon, for example, Amselle (2014) describes a shamanic tourism sector based on *ayahuasca* (a hallucinogenic beverage that causes visions). In this commodity chain, shamans are "entrepreneurs", "labeled healers" who advance "an indigenous ethnic identity [to] legitimize extensive knowledge in the field of traditional medicine and occupy a prominent place in the shamanic healing market". Tourists do not see themselves as such, but more as either patients or disciples in the process of initiation. Among them are patients (including terminal cancer and AIDS patients, for example) in search of remedies for all sorts of ailments, who, with regard to modern medicine, have tried everything without success. However, according to Amselle (2014), it is the healing of stress that constitutes the main business of the shamanic centers. Amselle even observes the building of alternative hospitals offering a wider range of treatments than just *ayahuasca* consumption and administered by what he calls "shaman operators". These centers are equipped with psychologists and doctors in order to gain legitimacy.

Indeed, this is the problem: legitimacy. In these trends of neo-shamanic and neo-traditional care, inherited knowledge (more or less rearranged in the 21st century fashion) and practices which resemble sectarian aberrations are, intertwined, as well as others which really resemble scams, praising "magical" substances that science has shown to be inoperative. Concerning *ayahuasca*, there are reports of non-consensual sexual relations imposed by shamans, as well as serious psychiatric disorders following the absorption of psychotropic drugs and even cases of death by cardiac arrest.

Amazonian shamanism based on *ayahuasca* is thus positioned between two diametrically opposed and incompatible visions. In France, organizers of trips to Amazonian centers have been prosecuted, notably for indoctrination, leading to the prohibition of *ayahuasca,* classified as a narcotic, in 2008. At the same time, the Peruvian government has declared the "authentic" use of *ayahuasca* as cultural heritage (Amselle 2014) and, according to Basset (2013),

> contrary to the classical approaches denouncing the ineluctable folklorization and cultural standardization of the receiving society, the process of idealization and commercialization of an Amerindian

> culture through tourism can give rise to cultural recognition among a wider public. Furthermore, it can lead to cultural revitalization from a local perspective and cultural diversification from a global perspective. In other words, shamanic or mystical-spiritual tourism destabilizes tradition while strengthening it.

Whether it is a matter of "opening the doors of perception" as A. Huxley wrote in 1954, or of a temporal psychotic decompensation (psychiatric designation), "it is always outside the beacons of reason that the experience is supposed to take shape" (Demanget 2015), and this is what, in terms of health, constitutes a strong limit to shamanic tourism. Since care in an altered state of consciousness benefits in some cases from recognition and scientific evidence (hypnosis is operated on in France according to certain medical indications), this requires a strict and rigorous control that does not exist in neo-shamanic tourism.

Fortunately, in a majority of cases, the call to nature and traditional and ancestral knowledge does not have great consequences in health, and at most, constitutes a pecuniary exploitation of the idealized dream of return to the sources of tourism.

In Mexico, on the Riviera Maya, from Cancún to Tulum via Playa del Carmen, there are numerous offers stamped with the "Mayan" label (see Figure 3.9). We asked a Canadian woman living on the coast and offering a mix of vegan naturopathic diets, yoga sessions and traditional Mayan massages, what documentation she had of her practice of traditional Mayan healing (written or transcribed from an oral transmission). She did not have any. A quick bibliographic search revealed that the Mayans do not really have a tradition of massage (except for breast massages intended to promote the rising of milk and diminish the pain of nursing mothers).

It is thus rather an exploitation of a current trend for tourism, based on a model that seems to have been imported from Asia where traditional massages proposed to tourists are legion. For the moment, it seems to be a niche market or an "oversale" (a complement sold in addition to a classic tourist service) to reinforce the attractiveness of the already existing hospitality. However, the trend seems to be towards development with resorts that specialize in well-being, backed by a discourse that highlights traditional health knowledge, for example, in Tulum, Mexico, around Mayan treatments; in Tarazoute, Morocco, around argan tree derivatives; in Bali around a holistic image of health, spirituality and nutrition. This phenomenon can also be seen in the west, particularly in France, through the revival of spa and thalassotherapy/balneotherapy facilities. It is then a question, for example, of connecting the thermal establishment to the neighboring salt marshes and putting forward the quartet of "care, well-being, nature and soil"!

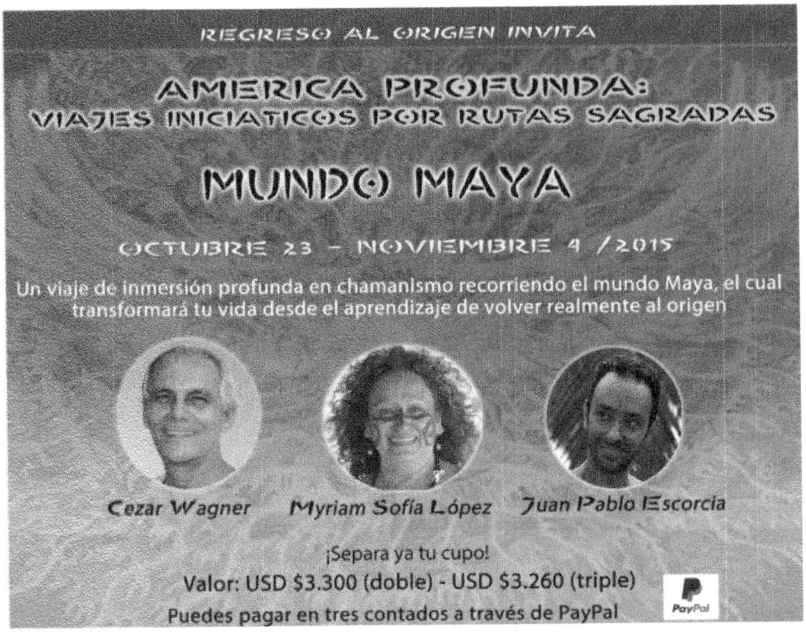

Figure 3.9. *Advertising for a Mayan shamanism initiation trip*

4

Impact of Tourism Development on the Health of Destinations

The decision to develop a geographic region through tourism activity implies that the region will be transformed on several levels. Infrastructures will have to be adapted (transportation, accommodation capacities and services, including health services) and the population will evolve, including a proportion of non-permanent residents who do not have the same needs as permanent residents. The labor market will also be impacted, as will, in varying degrees, the environment. This fourth chapter provides an overview of the various potential impacts of regional development through tourism activity, viewed through the prism of the health challenges, not for the tourists themselves, but for the local populations. These impacts can be grouped into three broad categories that will be successively addressed in the pages that follow: the impacts on health systems, the environmental impacts that constitute health challenges and, finally, the social and healthcare impacts.

4.1. Impacts on health systems

The presence of a population of tourists, temporary residents in a territory, is not without its effects on the health systems. These manifest themselves in several ways. First, the supply of care is modified in order to cater for the specific needs of this population (see Chapter 2). In particular, the question arises as to whether adapting the supply of healthcare to tourists unbalances local systems, especially where there is a strong difference in living standards between destinations and countries of origin, and where the risks involved in a two-tier healthcare system are significant. Second, the presence of tourists in a territory may make it necessary to implement public

For a color version of all the figures in this chapter, see www.iste.co.uk/fleuret/tourism.zip.

health policies, in particular, through prevention and awareness-raising actions around various risks. However, do these policies have a positive impact on local societies? Third, the development of tourism is accompanied by standards and accreditations, some of which have an impact on health and which may constitute a lever for action in favor of an overall improvement in the health of the territories. Finally, there is the question of the impact of a very specific type of tourism: medical tourism, which will draw resources and skills towards establishments that target an international clientele in countries where sometimes the basic supply of healthcare to the population is not yet guaranteed.

4.1.1. *Does tourism unbalance local health systems?*

The presence of tourists in a destination creates a need for infrastructure. There is no need to travel to exotic destinations to see the pressure that tourism puts on healthcare systems. The PACA (Provence-Alpes-Côte d'Azur) region provides a good example. On July 27, 2001, the French business daily *Les Echos* ran the headline: "Hospitals in tourist regions are overwhelmed". This article noted that, in the middle of the summer season and in addition to the chronic shortage of personnel in French hospitals, there are personnel on leave, which jeopardizes "the continuity and quality of the service to the public", particularly in coastal areas where, at the same time, the population is growing due to a large number of tourists (it is not unusual to see the population treble in certain places). The example of the emergency room at the Antibes-Juan-les-Pins Hospital Center (in the Alpes-Maritimes department of France) was given in the article: from an average of 70 admissions per day during the rest of the year, the number of increases to 150 per day between July 1 and August 15, and 100% of the short-stay beds are occupied. In addition, although credits are released to finance the replacement of personnel on vacation (limited to 15 days per person), those replacement positions are not being filled due to a lack of candidates. Some specialties are more complicated than others in terms of recruitment: in Antibes, for example, there is a shortage of radiology assistants. This issue of access to care can also be seen in the field of urban medicine, and yet, with 524.8 general practitioners per 100,000 inhabitants, the PACA region leads French regions in terms of medical density.

This is not an isolated example. In winter, in the French Alps, some resorts struggle to recruit seasonal doctors to cope with the influx of tourists, yet there are numerous ski accidents, which make it necessary to have sufficient medical care. A study by the Auvergne-Rhône-Alpes regional health observatory (2009[1]) on the tourist cantons of the Alpine ski area showed that, taking into account the population

1 Available at: http://www.ors-auvergne-rhone-alpes.org/pdf/Offredesoins_saisonniers_plaquette.pdf.

present in season, the medical density halves, falling from 11 doctors per 100,000 when calculated on the permanent population to 6 per 100,000 when tourists are included. During the winter and summer seasons, the activity of medical practices must also adapt to the increase in seasonal activity by extending opening hours, increasing the frequency of on-call duty, staggering vacations and compensating for the seasonal overactivity by long periods of inactivity out of season and mechanically reducing the supply of care available to the permanent population.

The problem becomes even more acute when we look at international tourism and observe the situation in Southern Hemisphere countries, where a two-tier health system may be observed, which is efficient and lucrative as a destination for tourists, but underdeveloped for the local population. This latter situation results from the fact that health professionals (such as nurses and doctors) may turn away from caring for local populations in favor of the more lucrative tourist trade (Lovel and Feuerstein 1992). Our field observations in Cancún, Mexico, for example, have enabled us to observe differences in fees for a general medical consultation ranging from 1 to 80 between a *Seguro Popular* ("Popular Security", a universal social insurance scheme) hospital and a private consulting room in one of the luxurious hotels in the hotel zone. This pricing differential has the effect of diverting health professionals away from the low-paying public sector to the private sector, with the result that healthcare facilities for the poorest local populations are underfunded. The difference in revenue linked to the difference in the price of consultations is also reflected in a difference in the equipment available and the hygiene standards introduced.

A study conducted specifically on medical tourism in Thailand showed that, through direct and indirect effects, medical tourism "exacerbates the shortage of medical personnel by diverting more and more workers from the private and public sectors to hospitals treating foreigners. This results in substantially higher costs in private hospitals and is likely to do the same for public hospitals and the universal health insurance system that covers most Thais" (NaRanong and NaRanong 2011).

In addition to the economic impact on the supply of healthcare, there are also indirect effects which are linked primarily to a change in the standard of living, which gives only some of the population access to other types of healthcare. Thus, the more affluent classes in the tourist region can now have access to more comfortable care. For example, a physiotherapist we met in Playa del Carmen told us, "The presence of tourists has two effects for me: a rise in the local cost of living creating an upper middle class that constitutes my privileged clientele, and, secondly, tourists are a source of clientele."

For authorities, being a jurisdiction that is very strong in tourism is an argument in budget discussions and requests for subsidies (Quintana Roo provides 30% of

Mexico's hard currency earnings, so the local authorities require a return of this value – 30% – from the Federal Government). For example, the overcrowded, obsolete and poorly located general hospital in Cancún was recently rebuilt and, according to a doctor there, "It was tourism that made it possible to have the money needed for construction; not because of the provision of services for tourists, but because tourism generates urban growth and population growth, and therefore new needs (including labor immigration into the tourist area)." According to the State Health Director, the presence of tourism is a benefit, especially for the general economy. For example, "The fact that a young state like Quintana Roo already has three major modern hospitals is due to tourism (see the 'impressive' hospital in Playa del Carmen); it is obvious to me that the state will participate in the development of health tourism in the near future."

Elsewhere, in Bali, for instance, the same cost differential can be observed between public hospitals for locals and clinics for tourists. However, local legislation requires doctors who provide private consultations in tourist clinics to provide an equivalent number of hours of consultations in the public sector, which allows a relative rebalancing and means that the tourist sector contributes to the local health system.

Another beneficial effect of tourism can be seen in Bali, particularly in the more rural and less densely populated north of the island: the increase in tourist numbers has generated a need for permanent care, and, as there is no hospital, this role is fulfilled by *puskesmas* (primary healthcare centers). For this, the centers had to be improved, as much in terms of equipment and skills (where before there was only a nurse or an assistant, there is now a complete medical team) as in terms of their opening hours, since all of them are now open 24 hours a day, 7 days a week.

A final notable impact in Bali is related to a tragic event: the bombings of October 12, 2002. Two bombs exploded in the tourist area of Kuta, killing 202 people and injuring 209 others. Most of the victims were foreign tourists, mainly Australian nationals (88 of whom died in this attack). The Australian authorities realized that Bali was a popular tourist destination for their nationals, but that it did not offer a full range of health services for them. It therefore became essential for Australia to integrate the health dimension into its bilateral cooperation program with Indonesia, since the level of health facilities in the tourist destination indirectly depends on the physical integrity of its citizens. Thus, several measures were enacted following the attack, the main ones being assistance in the purchase of hospital medical supplies, a grant to the Indonesian Red Cross, and a psychological assistance cell as an immediate response to the tragedy. In the longer term, the Australian government voted to provide A$10.5 million in assistance to the Balinese health system, including an investment in the Sanglah General Hospital in Denpasar in order to provide an intensive care unit and a medical training program worth A$3 million over five years. This example shows how health, which was initially not considered in tourism development, becomes central through a security concern and how, in the end, it is a country that sends tourists that intervenes in the healthcare system of a receiving country (Fleuret 2020). Of course, the Kuta bombing was an exceptional event, but, beyond the tragedy and its after-effects, Balinese health actors readily acknowledge that tourism has led to a rise in standards in hospitals (in Bali, the bombing accelerated this process) and even in dispensaries (*puskesmas*), some of which have developed a 24/7 service due to the presence of tourists, when the local population alone would not have justified such a service.

Elsewhere in the world, the same phenomenon can be observed: the needs of tourists generate investments in the health sector financed by the economic windfall that this sector represents. In Marrakech, for example, the new private hospital offers services that are equivalent or even superior to some European hospitals; but even while this hospital has a pricing policy that is accessible to the local population, this is not the case everywhere around the world.

Sometimes a healthcare service is set up for tourists, for example, a health center in an area that is suitable for scuba diving, which is essential in case of an accident. However, it is also possible that this does not benefit the local population at all, either because they do not have access to it or because they cannot afford the services.

The imbalance in living standards is also leading to the development of low-cost drug offers. In Latin America, and particularly in Mexico, *farmacias de ahoro* (low-cost pharmacies, Figure 4.1) are based on a simple concept: that the medical consultation is free but the patient pays for their medicines so the establishment pays itself on the prescription.

It is interesting to observe that some tourists, among the less fortunate, use these establishments. For them, the consultation costs 50 pesos (€2.50) and the prescriptions are paid. The doctor is paid for the consultation and receives a percentage on the medicines sold from their prescription. We tested it: the consultation lasts 2 minutes, watch in hand, and the waiting room is always full. Another type of pharmacy is only used by the local population (and a few adventurous tourists): the *farmacias similares*, whose slogan is *lo mismo pero mas barato* (the same, but cheaper) and where only generic drugs are sold, especially those from countries such as Brazil, South Africa and India.

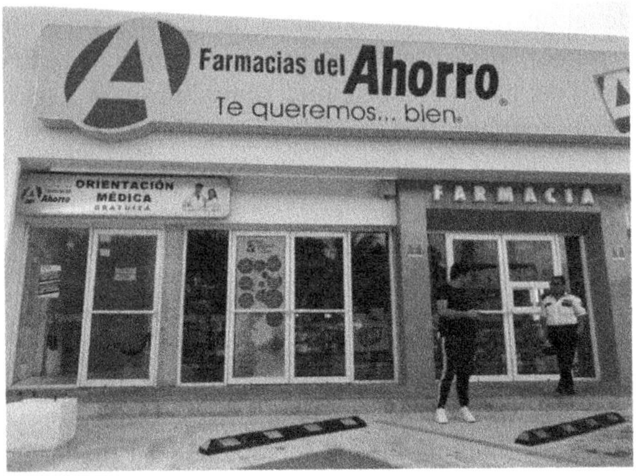

Figure 4.1. *Low-cost pharmacy in Mexico (photo: S. Fleuret 2017)*

These differences between pharmacies are a reminder that the process of accessing medicines varies widely around the world, as shown in Figure 4.2. Thanks to these three types of pharmacies, Mexico claims that over 90% of its population has access to essential medicines and vaccines. However, this is far from being the case everywhere, including in destinations where tourism exists but does not benefit the entire population of the area: in Tunisia and Morocco, for example, nearly a third of the population does not have access to essential medicines. In some other African countries, in India or in Brazil (although they produce generic medicines), this rate is over 50%.

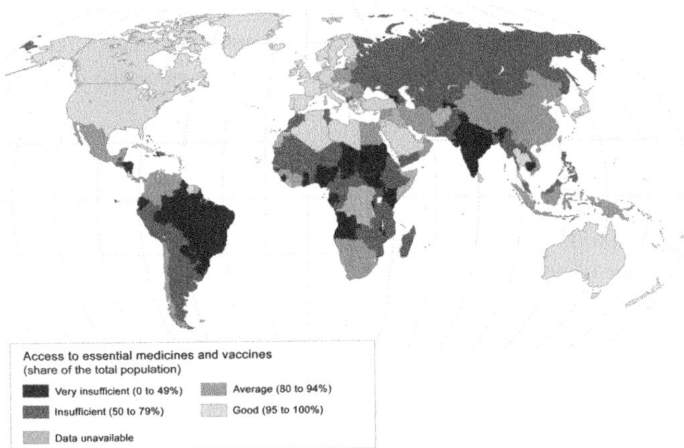

Figure 4.2. *Variations in access to medicines and vaccines around the world (source: UNDP, Human Development Report, 2004; background map: FNSP. Sciences Po – Cartography workshop CC BY 4.0; design and production: S. Fleuret, A. Lepetit, UMR 6590 ESO)*

However, even in places where access to healthcare for all is not guaranteed, it is possible for the tourist to access it for a fee or to be repatriated. The testimony reproduced below is based on a review left by a tourist on the *Tripadvisor* website (Figure 4.3). The experience of this tourist, who advises not going "just anywhere" but to a *Hospiten* establishment that is part of a chain of hospitals, originally located in the Balearic Islands and which has recently been established on the Riviera Maya, Mexico, raises a fundamental question that concerns the ethics of tourism.

Do the locals have the choice that this tourist had to select the facility that will provide them with safe and quality care? Evidently not. Therefore, it would certainly be appropriate to consider that, so long as this condition is not met, the development of the region through tourism is incomplete and must be (re)thought of differently. This reflection will be developed in Chapter 5.

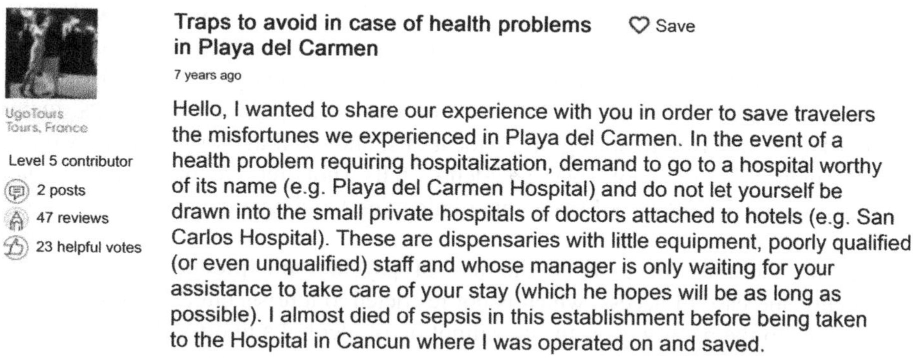

UgoTours
Tours, France
Level 5 contributor
2 posts
47 reviews
23 helpful votes

Traps to avoid in case of health problems in Playa del Carmen ♡ Save

7 years ago

Hello, I wanted to share our experience with you in order to save travelers the misfortunes we experienced in Playa del Carmen. In the event of a health problem requiring hospitalization, demand to go to a hospital worthy of its name (e.g. Playa del Carmen Hospital) and do not let yourself be drawn into the small private hospitals of doctors attached to hotels (e.g. San Carlos Hospital). These are dispensaries with little equipment, poorly qualified (or even unqualified) staff and whose manager is only waiting for your assistance to take care of your stay (which he hopes will be as long as possible). I almost died of sepsis in this establishment before being taken to the Hospital in Cancun where I was operated on and saved.

Figure 4.3. *Translated screenshot from the Tripadvisor website*

4.1.2. *Does tourism initiate public health policies?*

Scientific literature contains numerous writings on tourist behaviors and activities that may be risky for their health and/or that of local populations. For example, Sönmez et al. (2006) studied binge drinking and the risks associated with sexual activities during spring break in Cancún. This behavioral approach raises the more general healthcare challenges linked to tourism, as well as the question of whether the presence of tourists can initiate public health policies in this area. Among these, one specific policy that will be discussed later is occupational health. In the following pages, we will focus on the prevention of risks related to tourist behavior and the possible consequences for the local population, using two emblematic cases: risky behavior related to alcohol and drugs, and risks related to sexuality. We will then discuss the public health issues related to hygiene and water.

4.1.2.1. *Prevention of risky behaviors related to alcohol and drugs*

Spring break is a week-long vacation period during which young American students enjoy a week of often outrageous parties in tropical destinations within reasonable distance of the United States, in the Gulf of Mexico. Cancún is the emblematic destination for this phenomenon. Spring break is marked by the abuse of various substances (drugs and alcohol) in a context of collective disinhibition (Sönmez et al. 2006), where inebriation is frequently accompanied by unprotected sexual activity. In the authors' study, the main motivations for going on spring break were the possibility of drinking (78% of young men and 46% of young women), sex (74% and 31%, respectively) and experimenting with drugs (24% and 9%, respectively). Other main motivations cited were to escape stress and boredom (95% and 97%) and to find adventure (91% and 81%). At the end of their stay, 51% of young men and 39% of young women reported having being drunk and 21% of young men even reported passing out. Two-thirds of the respondents, with little difference by gender, reported having had unprotected sex (the survey did not say anything about drug use). In addition to the risk of sexually transmitted diseases during unprotected sex under the influence of alcohol or psychotropic drugs, many other risks are reported in spring break locations, and local authorities try in vain to prevent them: the risks of road accidents, falls (hoteliers report, for example, attempts to jump into the pool from upper balconies[2]) and, mainly, drownings.

Beyond the risk for tourists, the use of psychotropic products implies their availability and ease of access, which is not restricted to tourists but also exposes local populations to them. However, the consumption of alcohol and drugs by locals is not necessarily for festive purposes, but rather as a palliative to their difficult living conditions. In Mexico, this problem is compounded by issues related to drug trafficking. Drug dealers have a strong influence on the local society, which is plagued by violence and racketeering (*derecho de piso*[3], imposed on dealers)…

Through excesses, the tourist participates indirectly and very involuntarily and can, in turn, suffer the consequences if the destination becomes unsafe. Acapulco, on the Pacific coast, is a tragic illustration: this coastal city has gone from being a dream resort to a very dangerous city, which causes tourists to flee and creates a vicious circle of disaffection and worsening social problems against a backdrop of drug trafficking. The authorities are aware of the problem and are struggling to curb this phenomenon, the roots of which are probably in public health policies, which should be coordinated with those of the sending countries, whose youth are relocating their excesses. For example, one of the reasons why young Americans go to Mexico

2 Practice called "balconing" that is found in other destinations, especially in the Balearic Islands, and has significant repercussions for hospital emergency services.

3 Right of door step.

is the possibility of drinking alcohol from the age of 18, as opposed to 21 in their own country.

4.1.2.2. *Risks related to sexuality*

Another famous place for party tourism is Thailand and, in particular, the Khosan Road area of Bangkok. During the emergence of the HIV-AIDS pandemic, this was one of the first places to study the relationship between tourism, sexuality and health risks (Cohen 1988).

Public health policies must come from the government, which is often problematic for a variety of reasons, including the fear of exposing a phenomenon that would scare away tourists and the financial windfall. In Thailand, it appears that HIV has not had a direct impact on tourist numbers. This is, therefore, a problem linked to the local population: HIV does not threaten the tourist industry, but the health of the country's inhabitants. Thailand is a good example of how governments have had to rethink their tourism policy and include a public health policy to prevent the risk of HIV-AIDS. In the 1980s,

> prostitutes working with foreign tourists were quickly identified as being responsible for the introduction and spread of the virus in the country, and tourism, long praised for its developmental virtues, suddenly appeared to be a threat to the very survival of society. Repressive projects multiplied (such as blood tests for tourists and sanatoria for prostitutes), testifying to the feverishness and sense of urgency that seized the political and administrative authorities (Roux 2008).

The first reaction of the authorities was therefore an authoritarian and coercive reflex in an effort to stop the spread of the virus. Prostitutes were stigmatized and became culpable for the transmission of the virus contracted from tourists to the indigenous population. However, at the same time, the tourist industry continued to require that the movement of tourists be free and that the country not be designated as "infested by the virus" (an unfortunate expression from the Minister of Health in 1989): "The attractiveness of prostitution establishments is not foreign to the success of the kingdom" (Roux 2008). The 1991 coup d'état marked a fundamental change in Thai AIDS management with the implementation of a massive prevention policy promoting the systematic use of condoms. The fight against discrimination against the sick was also initiated, in cooperation with NGOs fighting against HIV. Thus, measures have targeted attitudes and behavior by aiming to encourage, for example, "marital fidelity, [the] public commitment of Thai men (especially in the north, one of the regions most affected by the virus) to refuse prostitutes, [the] media stance against the supposed sexual licentiousness of youth" (Roux 2008). At the same time, sex tourism and sex tours were denounced and "normal" tourism was encouraged.

Since then, "it is no longer the tourist who is designated as the importer of the disease, but the sex tourist"; the virus is specified and the risk defined.

4.1.2.3. *Hygiene, water and public health in tourist destinations*

In countries of the Southern Hemisphere, there is also an area in which international programs exist that are examples of positive conjunction, and lead to a virtuous circle. Earlier in this book, we mentioned the WASH (Water Sanitation and Hygiene)[4] program by developing the example of Madagascar. This United Nations program collectively addresses water, sanitation and hygiene issues, key issues that are grouped together due to their interdependent nature, although each represents a separate field of action. For example, without toilets, water sources are contaminated; without clean water, basic hygiene is impossible. Tourism can, in some situations, contribute to the implementation of public health policies related to water, sanitation and hygiene, and the WASH program provides a framework for implementation. This was the case in the Philippines, for example, on Masbate Island, where poor hygiene and unsanitary conditions contrasted with the beauty of the area and, especially, the beaches, which were very attractive for tourism (Figure 4.4).

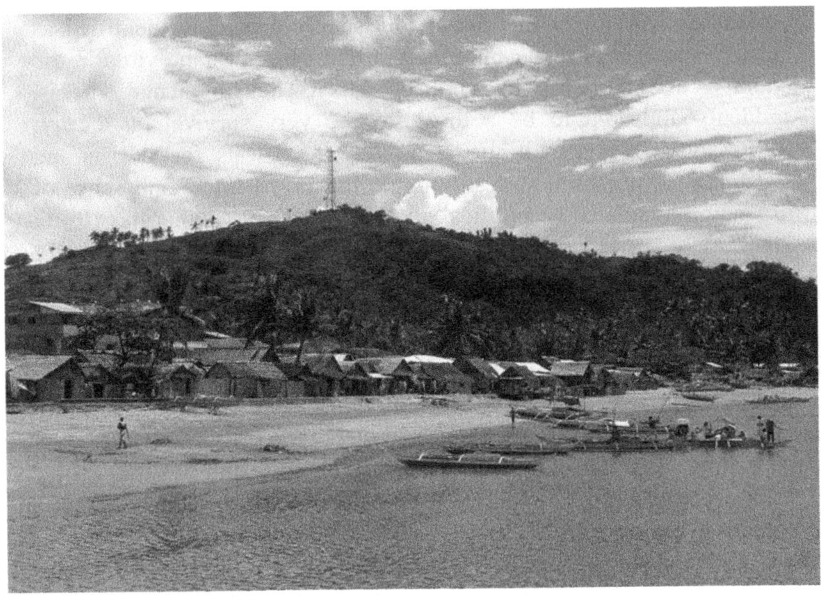

Figure 4.4. *Masbate, Philippines (photo: J. Beaulieu, Flickr)*

4 See section 2.1.1.3: "Orofecal infections and risks related to water, sanitation and hygiene (WASH)".

> Previously, we had a problem with tourism because most of our people practice open defecation, especially on the beaches. We have beautiful beaches, but they are very dirty. When the WASH program came to our municipality, cleanliness and hygiene were introduced: we encouraged everyone to build their own toilets, and, because water is also a problem, we simultaneously implemented water and sanitation projects. The WASH program has had a big impact in our municipality because we have reduced the share of water-related infectious diseases, and, at the same time, our population has been educated about cleanliness and the importance of drinking safe water (Arturo Virtucio of Aroroy, Mayor of Masbate[5]).

Through this example, we understand how tourism, through the standards it conveys, especially in terms of hygiene and access to water, can be a driver for change with an impact on health.

In many places, access to water is a crucial issue and while in the previous example tourism had a positive influence, it can also have a negative impact, as in Bali, which is experiencing a serious crisis related to the pressure exerted on the water resource by the influx of tourists in this tropical destination. However, the island is endowed with water resources in the north which, combined with rich volcanic soils, allows for a flourishing agriculture. Yet population growth, coupled with the expansion of tourism (3.8 million residents and 2.7 million tourists in 2011), has ultimately put a strain on this resource and it is now estimated that 60% of the island's watersheds are dried up[6]. Imported western lifestyles and the development of infrastructure for tourists (villas, hotels, swimming pools, spas, etc.) explain this crisis. While a native consumes an average of 30 to 50 liters per day, a tourist consumes between 150 and 200 liters. It is estimated that the tourism sector consumes 65% of the water resources in Bali. In addition to the scarcity of the resource that is available for agriculture, this has consequences on the environment and, indirectly, on the health of the population. As runoff water is less abundant, it has higher concentrations of pollutants from excess agricultural inputs (used to produce more in order to meet the demand of tourism) and contamination from unregulated landfills (where waste is, again, largely the result of tourism). Thus, in Bali, wells that do not dry up contain water that is unfit for consumption. The local authorities have set up a plan, the Bali Water Program, to try to remedy this problem, which involves the construction of retention basins to create water reserves, and campaigns to raise awareness of water consumption. Here, we find the issue of the ethics of tourism development that have already been mentioned. The most advanced hotels on this subject have, for example, set up water recycling systems to reuse gray water from

5 Available at: https://www.watergovernance.org/programmes/goal-wash/philippines/.

6 Available at: https://exofoundation.org/bali-water-crisis/.

toilets, for instance, or to operate their pools, spas and other jacuzzis in a closed circuit. Raising awareness among tourists is essential to encourage all stakeholders to move towards more virtuous practices, and this can be achieved through the development of labels – or accreditations – and certifications

4.1.3. *Labels and certification standards*

Tourists go in search of an experience that is free of defects and constraints. Vacation time is dedicated to rest and relaxation; nevertheless, a significant proportion of tourists are ready to direct their choices towards an offer of eco-responsible or socially responsible products. Health is not yet a sufficiently conscious concern for determining choices, except on one point: hygiene and safety in the face of the risk of infection. For these parameters, there are labels and certifications that guarantee to tourist facility clientele that these facilities respect norms that conform to western standards. These are important levers that can be activated by the issuers (tour operators) and tourists who, in an ideal world, should be better informed and demand them. For the recipients (hoteliers, restaurant owners, etc.), it is sometimes a challenge to obtain and display a label in order to attract new customers or to obtain a quality certification or an additional star.

To date, there is no global "healthy tourism" label, but the violence of the impact of the Covid-19 crisis gives some hope of an awareness that may allow such a label to be created (see below). In the meantime, health is a parameter for which a few rare indicators are disseminated in the specifications of various labels. It only constitutes a label in its own right in the field of medical tourism. Some labels are presented below.

4.1.3.1. *Concerning hygiene*

Distintivo H (the "H" here stands for "Hygiene") is a Mexican government program that aims to reduce the incidence of food-borne diseases and, at the same time, improve the image of Mexico as a tourist destination. Therefore, this certification is issued by the Ministry of Tourism. There are national equivalents in many tourist destinations and these awards are interesting because they condition the whole chain. Distintivo H comprises of 135 control criteria that cover the different stages of food and beverage distribution, such as food reception, storage, product handling, refrigeration and freezing (equipment and cold chain management), kitchen and bar areas, food preparation, service areas, water and ice, employee sanitary facilities, waste management and hygiene practices.

For example, an incoming food item should never cross paths with an outgoing food item in the kitchen. This means that the dock and delivery lanes leading to the storage area and cold stores are different from the exit lanes and the garbage collection dock. This means that kitchens have to be adapted and an investment is often required to adapt the premises if they are not built directly to standard.

The *ISO 22000 standard* is a certification that proves a company's ability to ensure food safety throughout the food chain. It is an international standard and is linked to ISO 9001 (quality management) and ISO 14001 (environmental management). The ISO 22000 standard deals with hygiene and good practices at all stages of the process, as does Distintivo H, the difference being that it is an international certification that is consistent across all countries.

4.1.3.2. *Concerning well-being*

WellHotel is a certification that focuses on wellness and targets three types of customers: wellness tourists (such as spa customers), business tourists looking for relaxation after work and tourists that are recovering from illness. WellHotel offers three levels of certification based on a predefined program called Standard Operating Procedures (SOP). Obtaining this label assumes that different standards of equipment, comfort, hygiene, services, level of training of staff and professionals and so on are controlled. Each level (for a fee, of course) entitles the holder to targeted communication campaigns by the certifying body in specific magazines, brochures and sales sites. For example, obtaining Level 3 entitles, in addition to the WellHotel certification, access to two webcasts for prospecting and developing customer loyalty, five training courses delivering a "wellness travel" professional certificate, a marketing campaign on LinkedIn, a full-page advertisement in three magazines (*Corporate Wellness Magazine*, *Luxury Hoteliers Magazine* and *Medical Tourism Magazine*) and monthly campaigns on social networks to promote the establishment.

This example illustrates the intertwining of the development of wellness components and commercial promotion issues.

4.1.3.3. *Concerning security*

Safe Hotel Executive is a label that covers, for example, safety, firefighting equipment, evacuation and staff training in risk management. Certification via this label covers a total of 222 standardization points and three levels: standard, executive and premium, for those who perform beyond the required standards.

4.1.3.4. *Concerning health*

Joint Commission International (JCI) is a monitoring and accreditation body for healthcare facilities that verifies compliance with standards in clinics and hospitals. Since it is an American structure, the reference standards are those of the United States. In the medical tourism industry, facilities seek JCI certification because it allows them to guarantee safety and gain the trust of patients. However, this is also an issue for local hospitals or large chains of private healthcare facilities that are located in tourist areas (such as Hospiten).

In 2020, all countries around the world were affected by the Covid-19 pandemic: some experienced large numbers of cases and had to confine their populations for varying lengths of time. Other countries were less affected (notably in Africa), but the lockdown of populations in the sending countries had the effect of drying up the flow of tourists. Faced with this crisis and the scarcity of tourists, hoteliers reacted and are now displaying health information on their communication media to reassure their customers. At the time of this crisis, a study was already underway to analyze how health and well-being were positioned in the communications of hotels of the Riviera Maya in Mexico, through their websites. The results speak for themselves: before the emergence of the pandemic, the presence of health facilities or sanitary standards was either not used or hardly used as a commercial argument, and only wellness in the sense of "rest, relaxation and self-care" was displayed as a "plus" by the most luxurious hotels, with this announcement rarely on the home page. However, immediately after the crisis broke, the websites of these hotels changed: all, without exception, now display their list of anti-Covid precautions. Principal among these is the Safe Guest program, which guarantees, for instance, the disinfection of rooms and common areas and the respect of various social distancing measures. Search engines and booking sites such as Booking.com or Tripadvisor also now prominently display hygiene and public health measures taken in the face of the coronavirus disease (Figure 4.5).

This is a question of reassuring the client in a pandemic context, which demonstrates that health, normally relatively ignored in the context of tourism, can suddenly become a priority in the event of a crisis.

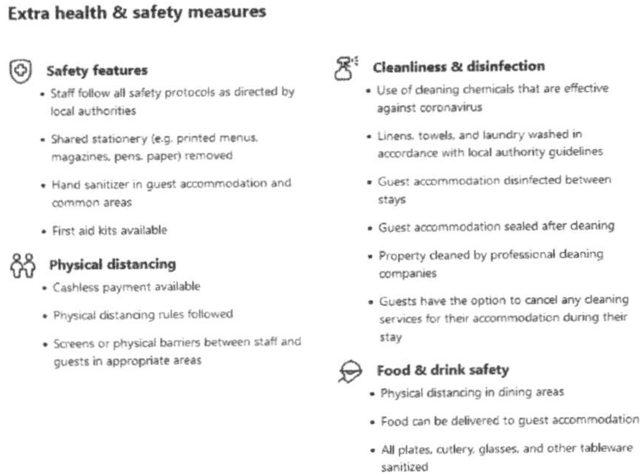

Extra health & safety measures

Safety features
- Staff follow all safety protocols as directed by local authorities
- Shared stationery (e.g. printed menus, magazines, pens, paper) removed
- Hand sanitizer in guest accommodation and common areas
- First aid kits available

Physical distancing
- Cashless payment available
- Physical distancing rules followed
- Screens or physical barriers between staff and guests in appropriate areas

Cleanliness & disinfection
- Use of cleaning chemicals that are effective against coronavirus
- Linens, towels, and laundry washed in accordance with local authority guidelines
- Guest accommodation disinfected between stays
- Guest accommodation sealed after cleaning
- Property cleaned by professional cleaning companies
- Guests have the option to cancel any cleaning services for their accommodation during their stay

Food & drink safety
- Physical distancing in dining areas
- Food can be delivered to guest accommodation
- All plates, cutlery, glasses, and other tableware sanitized

Figure 4.5. *Excerpt from Booking.com, 02/03/2021*

4.1.4. *Special case: the impact of medical tourism*

If there is one area in which the impacts on health and healthcare systems in destinations have been studied, it is medical tourism (Johnston et al. 2010). On January 1, 2018, the online media outlet *Slate.fr* ran the headline "*Les hôpitaux indiens sont remplis d'Américains désespérés*" (Indian Hospitals Are Filled With Desperate Americans), and questioned under the subheading whether medical tourists with deep pockets were the cause of the healthcare system's problems or even their cure[7].

4.1.4.1. *A critical look at medical tourism*

Medical tourism must be observed with a critical eye (Crooks et al. 2010), particularly when it involves patients from so-called "developed" countries using the infrastructure of so-called "developing" countries. The question raised is that of the provision of health and care infrastructures for people who can afford these services and which may otherwise be inaccessible to citizens of the country concerned. Another ethical issue is the quality of care, when international patients are observed to receive a higher standard of care than local populations. Another critical issue is the training of medical personnel: very often this training is provided by publicly funded organizations (such as universities), and when graduates of these training programs are directed towards a professional practice that serves an international patient base and not a local one, we are entitled to ask whether investment in this training may not constitute a misuse of public funds. An alternative consideration is that surgeons from developing countries, who usually practice in facilities with low levels of equipment, may, within the framework of medical tourism, have access to and train with high-tech western standard equipment and thus participate in an overall rise in the competence of the country's medical personnel.

4.1.4.2. *Medical tourism as a source of income*

Medical tourism is a source of foreign currency for destination countries, but is subject to significant variations between countries and is particularly difficult to quantify (Johnston et al. 2010). Estimates vary widely depending on the sources: the number of Americans traveling abroad for care is estimated to be between 50,000 and 500,000 (Leahy 2008). With such an imprecise range, it is impossible to estimate the overall costs. Nevertheless, a report published by the Tourism Research and Marketing Group estimates that there are approximately 37 million health-related trips worldwide each year, which would generate a global revenue of approximately €33 billion (TRAM 2006). In 2015, a study by France Stratégie (Marguerit and Reynaudi) estimated the global medical tourism market at €60 billion. Despite the uncertainties about the value of financial flows generated, everyone agrees that this sector is growing rapidly. For low- and medium-development countries,

7 Available at: http://www.slate.fr/story/156281/inde-tourisme-medical-systeme-sante-hopitaux.

Johnston et al. (2010) estimate the growth potential at 25% per year, and Menvielle and Menvielle (2013) refer to a "global supermarket" of medical tourism.

In addition, medical tourists "are particularly attractive because they inject more cash into the local economy compared with traditional tourists. For example, it has been estimated that medical tourists who travel to Asia spend more than twice as much as traditional tourists" (Johnston et al. 2010). This cash can, in an ideal world, be re-injected into the local health system, as is the case in Cuba, according to Charatan (2001).

4.1.4.3. *Can medical tourism contribute to the improvement of healthcare systems?*

According to Crooks et al. (2010), with appropriate regulation, medical tourism can be "a valuable means by which developing countries can increase revenues and reduce bottlenecks in their health systems". The key word here is regulation. For example, a common criticism of medical tourism is that it can divert health professionals away from serving their populations. Indeed, the price differences between a procedure intended for the local population and a one intended for wealthy tourists can be colossal. Consequently, there is a risk that doctors will choose an international rather than a local patient base. However, Crooks et al. argue that the presence of international tourists in hospitals can reduce the "brain drain" that results from the fact that many surgeons, for example, leave to practice abroad, fleeing countries with poor health facilities. By justifying the presence of high-tech hospital equipment and international standard working environments, medical tourism structures contribute to the retention of medical personnel. With proper regulation, these skills can benefit both tourists and local populations: in Bali, for example, any doctor who practices on tourists must donate an equivalent amount of time to the local population within the Balinese system. This is a good example of regulation.

Other arguments are also put forward to defend the potentially positive impact of medical tourism. According to Herrick (2007), there may be a positive impact in the sending countries: the delocalization of care and thus the reduction in the number of patients in the national system may exert a competitive pressure to lower healthcare costs. For Lunt et al. (2011), medical tourism can encourage economies to maximize their comparative advantages in terms of labor costs, technology and capacity. However, these approaches are based on a very neoliberal view of the market economy, which is subject to many reservations because health is a very specific market.

Moreover, not all countries and health systems are necessarily conducive or adapted to the development of medical tourism. The France Stratégie study (Marguerit and Reynaudi 2015), for example, inventoried what would be needed for France to be able to develop this sector of activity. According to the authors,

> France, which does not lack assets, is struggling to position itself in this market. Certain fears have not been entirely dispelled, such as fears of two-tier medicine, of less access to care, and doubts about the real economic benefits. In fact, we must be careful not to see this source of financing as a solution to the financial difficulties of certain establishments and to budget cuts. The stakes are no less high: in addition to the direct economic benefits for the health sector, tourism, the science industry and construction, there are indirect benefits linked to France's influence strategy (increased research partnerships, international prestige, and so on).

According to this strategic note, in order to develop medical tourism in France, it is necessary to both "organize the arrival of foreign patients in the country", which is not self-evident, and "promote the influence of the French healthcare system abroad", while at the same time "preserving the values of the French healthcare system and improving the services provided to the insured".

Since France cannot claim any real competitive advantage in terms of costs over Southern Hemisphere countries, its strategic positioning should be based on the quality of the care provided. In fact, some French hospitals, particularly in oncology, are world-renowned. Another advantage is that waiting lists in France are relatively short, even while the situation has been deteriorating in recent years. Another report (Mantion and Peton 2011) highlights France's international reputation in terms of health aid and cooperation.

Finally, France is the world's leading tourist destination in terms of tourist flows and has all the necessary infrastructures in this area, whether in terms of hotel capacity, transport accessibility (particularly by air) or activities related to health and well-being (such as thalassotherapy).

Despite these advantages, the France Stratégie report estimates that there are only 8,900 foreign patients per year, or less than 0.1% of all admissions to medicine, surgery and obstetrics. The potential therefore seems to be largely under-used. In response to this observation, initiatives have been launched. French Health Care, for example, is a government-launched association designed to be an accreditation to federate and animate the network of healthcare actors and as an instrument for collective promotion on the international stage[8]. The challenge is to attract a high-end clientele and generate economic benefits, while also bringing cash into the largely

8 Available at: https://frenchhealthcare-association.fr/.

deficient French healthcare system. According to France Stratégie, hospitals should be organized in order to meet the expectations of non-resident patients, without jeopardizing the principle of equal access to care and the quality of treatment, and to offer complementary services to care, such as managing the preparation of the stay (visas, transportation, etc.), ensuring patient follow-up before and after medical procedures (such as translation services and post-operative follow-up) and responding to requests for quotes within tight deadlines. However, while some examples have made the headlines (see Box 4.1), overall medical tourism is struggling to develop within an unsuitable system in terms of pricing and reception procedures. This is a long way from the vision of medical tourism being able to bolster the coffers of the national healthcare system.

"We must stop rehashing the fantasy of an emir reserving a wing of the hospital to the detriment of French patients!" Jean-Patrick Lajonchère, Director General of the Paris-Saint Joseph Hospital Group, who in 2016 was tasked with a mission to promote French medical excellence internationally by the Ministry of Foreign Affairs, defends his business. The story he refers to is a little dated, but it made a lasting impression. In May 2014, a member of the Saudi Arabian royal family privatized nine rooms at Ambroise-Paré Hospital (AP-HP) in Boulogne-Billancourt, France, to house his bodyguards, reserved seven parking spaces, had showerheads installed in the toilets and had catered meals delivered.

"This high priced hospitalization – €270,000, according to *Le Canard Enchaîné* – had discredited the embryonic market for welcoming foreign patients" [...]

"Dozens of medical concierge or facilitating agencies had positioned themselves in this niche to organize stays, hotels and transportation, but the bubble quickly burst," admits Elie Moarbes, CEO of the Medical Tourism Network. "French doctors are still too cautious, believing that health is not a product like any other, and the French style of organization is still very complex, especially to obtain a quote or a visa." Meanwhile, Germany, Switzerland, the Netherlands and the United Kingdom have no qualms about courting this patient base.

Box 4.1. *Excerpt from "Challenges" magazine, 06/30/2020*

In addition, the Covid-19 crisis has stopped international flows and totally mobilized health systems on the care of patients affected by coronavirus, postponing the hypothetical development of medical tourism in France indefinitely.

4.2. Health and environmental impacts

As early as 1980, an OECD report pointed out the impacts of tourism on the environment and noted, among other things, that "on the one hand, a quality environment is essential for the practice of tourism, and, on the other, the quality of the environment is seriously threatened by the development of tourism itself". At the time, there was no talk of sustainable development (the Brundtland report, which was the first to popularize the term, was not published until 1987). However, seven years earlier, the OECD report had already noted that the environment is a "perishable asset" and listed the impacts of tourism by category, including: pollution (air, water, noteworthy sites, etc.), reduction of natural and agricultural areas, threats to fauna and flora, landscape degradation, congestion, saturation and conflicts. However, the report did not directly mention the health issues related to the environmental impacts of tourism, which we will detail below.

4.2.1. *Pollution or degradation of ecosystems*

4.2.1.1. *Water, coastlines, aquatic spaces and wetlands*[9]

Tourism impacts terrestrial and marine aquatic spaces in various ways: through wastewater that is, to an extent, treated and therefore polluted to varying degrees in the vicinity of tourist facilities, as well as, for example, through the contamination of water by boats (such as cruise ships).

A Turkish study (Kocasoy 1989) analyzed water pollution (the presence of coliform bacteria) in relation to a health questionnaire for tourists. Not surprisingly, the results showed that tourists who bathed near areas of sewage discharge into the sea suffered from gastrointestinal disorders more frequently than others, and, depending on their origin and age, tourists were prone to health disorders in varying degrees. Thus, Scandinavians and children were more affected, and the author hypothesized a lower immunity. Standards have evolved since then[10], but the conclusions of this study remain valid for many tourist destinations: "Any tourism development without the necessary pollution control infrastructures (in particular wastewater treatment) inevitably leads to pollution of the seas, with negative effects on human health. In this context, an uncontrolled increase in the number of tourists will have harmful, rather than positive effects both from an environmental and health point of view."

The pressure on the water resource is thus manifested in other ways than by pollution, such as through the over-extraction of the resource, either to supply hotels that consume a lot of water or to irrigate crops to feed the population that is growing with tourism. This over-extraction can have health impacts, by impeding access to water for local populations or by causing concentrations of toxic substances (such as pesticide residues) in over-subscribed water tables. In a study conducted in Latin

9 See also section 4.1.2, where water management in Bali is discussed from a public health policy perspective.

10 On this subject, see: https://gisposidonie.osupytheas.fr/ ?p=2093 [accessed 02/08/2021].

America (Stonich 1998), a political ecology approach was used to examine the relationship between tourism development, water and the health of the islands in the Gulf of Honduras. This study demonstrated that arable land, freshwater and seawater resources are compromised by uncontrolled tourism development and that the observed degradation is linked to power relations: the interests of the tourism industry take precedence over the interests of local populations through the relative power of control over water resources held by this sector. This results in unequal distribution and water quality and has impacts on ecological health. The study also demonstrated that poor mestizo immigrants and poor Afro-Caribbean residents are the most vulnerable to the ecological health risks from these activities.

The environmental impact of tourism has repercussions on fauna and flora and therefore indirectly on humans who, for example, consume seafood. Recently, the pollution linked to plastic waste has been headline news, through the identification of a vast vortex of floating plastic particles in the middle of the ocean over an area that is equivalent to three times the size of France and with a total estimated weight of 80,000 tonnes, resulting from the agglomeration, between two waters, of more than 1,800 billion micro-wastes (Lebreton et al. 2018). However, this pollution is located far from the coast and has little impact on tourism. In contrast, other similar pollutions have had much greater repercussions and impacts on the tourism sector: in March 2018, a diver uploaded a video onto YouTube in which he was seen swimming in a sea that was overrun by plastic waste[11]. This video was viewed more than 1,340,000 times, stirring the threat of tourist clientele fleeing and which seems to be driving stakeholders to mobilize to seek solutions and change behavior. Indonesia is the world's second largest producer of marine waste after China, with 1.29 million tonnes per year dumped at sea, causing immense damage to ecosystems and health (many types of waste can cause injuries and infections to bathers). The Indonesian government has committed to reducing marine plastic waste by 70% by 2025. It intends to increase recycling of litter, which is almost non-existent at the moment, launch clean-up campaigns and reduce the use of plastic bags in retail outlets. However, this will probably not be enough. On the beaches of northern Bali, in addition to the plastic bags in question, there are tubes of toothpaste, shampoo, sunscreen, bags of candy and more. On the beaches of Pemalang, to the north of the island, 700 cleaning employees and 35 trucks collect about 100 tons of garbage on the beaches every day to dump them in a nearby landfill. The next day, the situation is the same. The problem becomes worse during the rainy season, from November to March, when strong winds and marine currents carry the garbage onto the beaches and flooded rivers carry it to the coast.

11 Available at: https://www.20minutes.fr/planete/2232835-20180306-video-bali-plongeur-filme-milieu-ocean-dechets-plastiques.

Bali is particularly exposed, because of marine currents, but a growing number of coastal tourist areas are affected and the phenomenon, contrary to general public awareness, is not a new one. In 1996, Gardinier had already made a clear statement about the island of Malta: "Litter on beaches is a major problem for the management of coastal resources. A number of Maltese beaches have unsightly piles of litter, including plastic containers and objects such as freezers. There are used hypodermic needles, sanitary napkins and condoms, all of which causes health risks and can lead to damage to ecosystems."

Coastal areas are not alone in being concerned: rivers and lakes are also affected. In the Walloon Region, tourism represents an important sector of economic activity, particularly in the Ardennes, which is the second largest tourist area in Belgium (after the coast). Fishing and kayaking in the rivers and lakes attract many summer visitors. However, these leisure activities require a welcoming environment, if possible, preserved from any form of pollution. One study, carried out at the request of the Walloon Region (Rosillon et al. 2002), showed the interest in a broader approach, leading to a protection and a global management of the aquatic environments concerned, considering that a "poor quality of surface waters in tourism areas would inevitably lead to the loss of a significant potential for recreation and local tourism. Improving or preserving the quality of these waters is becoming a necessity, both from the point of view of human health and local development". The study therefore suggested the establishment and monitoring of area profiles, integrating the upstream part of the watercourse, the impact of the various activities in the basin and the degree of survival of pathogens in the natural environment, to enable integrated management (reinforced by the participation of various stakeholders) in order to achieve good surface water quality status. This example, like the previous, illustrates how tourism activities can be drivers of change in improving the environment and health in areas where recreational activities are practiced.

4.2.1.2. *Atmospheric pollution and other nuisances "in the air"*

This type of pollution, in relation to the tourism sector, is essentially caused by modes of transport, including the release of polluting particles by fossil fuel engines and noise pollution near airports or roads, as well as in the heart of natural areas. In Quebec, for example, certain lakes bordered by holiday homes impose regulations prohibiting motorized navigation in order to provide a true area for rest.

Pollution, health and tourism can be seen from two angles: the impact of pollution on the health of travelers on the one hand, and the impact of pollution generated by tourist flows on local populations on the other.

Regarding the health of travelers, a study conducted in Beijing, China, by Zhang et al. (2015) provides an interesting insight. The results of this study reveal that while potential tourists are relatively familiar with air pollution (on a scale of 1 to 5, their average knowledge is 2.76), this value rises to 4.58 out of 5 when asked about their awareness of the health risks of air pollution. However, this has little impact on their choice of tourist destinations, and the authors of the study believe that tourists passively accept the information they receive in the media about spikes in pollution levels. Another study (Sun et al. 2019), also focusing on China and specifically on domestic tourism, found that less than one percent of tourists consider that a pollution spike at their destination would have no or little impact on their trip. The impact of pollution is therefore potentially very strong, but it manifests itself differently depending on the purpose of the trip: tourists looking for landscapes and leisure activities are those who declare themselves to be the most impacted, while business tourists are much less concerned.

Another study, this time in Hong Kong, presented differences in perception depending on the geographical origin of the tourists. Asian tourists show a greater awareness of air pollution issues than westerners, "which contradicts the conventional wisdom that the latter pay more attention to air quality than the former" (Cheung and Law 2001). The study by Zhang et al. (2015) also compared the location of air pollution in tourists' choices with seven traditional factors that impact travelers (cost, distance, travel time, travel companions, safety, available products and destination popularity). This comparison shows that while pollution is still less important in destination choices and travel decisions than other criteria, it still has a strong impact and is a major secondary criterion. Indeed, despite their small proportion, a small number of tourists in the sample studied declared that they would consider changing their plans in the case of a pollution spike. More generally, they would postpone the dates of a trip to Beijing rather than cancel it. Finally, Zhang and his co-authors believe that pollution spikes and the health fears they cause among potential tourists impact the timing of arrivals: "In other words, air pollution plays an important role in the seasonality of tourism."

The potential health impacts of pollution of major urban tourism destinations are indeed significant. According to a study by the Transport & Environment NGO, tourists are affected by air pollution. The organization evaluated air pollution in the 10 most popular cities for tourists. According to its results, a short stay of four days in Paris would be the equivalent of having smoked two cigarettes[12]: the comparison is debatable, but its aim is, above all, to impress on the public the health risks of air pollution. The cause is clearly the high temperatures (here we find the seasonality) which lead to an increase in ozone pollution levels (for which the vehicles running on fossil fuels are primarily responsible). Unfortunately, the French capital is far from being alone in this case: Amsterdam, Rome and Vienna have the same bad results. To breathe easier, you have to fly to Dublin or Barcelona, where, for the same

12 Available at: https://www.transportenvironment.org/discover/summer-tourists-forced-smoke-top-european-cities/.

amount of time, the pollution rate is equivalent to one smoked cigarette. In this ranking, two cities are to be avoided, Prague and Istanbul, where the lungs are exposed as if smoking four cigarettes. However, why is the tourist more exposed than the simple city dweller who experiences the same pollution on a daily basis? Jens Müller, author of the study, explains that "when air pollution is bad, we are told to avoid eating or exercising outside. But walking around cities and eating on restaurant terraces is what city breaks are all about."

Preserving air quality is therefore a health issue but can also be a potential argument for tourist attractiveness, or repulsion. Tourist cities like Paris, Prague or Istanbul have to be concerned about this.

4.2.1.3. *Impacts on fauna and flora and health implications*

Air and noise pollution, water pollution, deforestation for the construction of infrastructures, over-frequentation of natural areas and so on have multiple impacts, ranging from disturbance of fauna to a decrease in biodiversity.

Human settlements in tourist and recreational areas are never neutral, even while, for several decades, particular attention has been paid to the sustainability of these settlements and attempts have been made to minimize their impact. The subject merits a book of its own, as the ramifications and indirect effects are many and often underestimated. Indeed, "The relationship between human health and biodiversity are complex [and] biodiversity can represent a threat to health, but health and human well-being also benefit from many services [through] the role of ecosystems in the regulation of diseases, pollution and the role of Nature in human well-being" (the French Foundation for Biodiversity Research[13]), which makes it an interdisciplinary subject (architecture, urban planning, ecology, geography, public health, etc.).

The One Health initiative, supported by the WHO (World Health Organization), the UN (United Nations), the FAO (Food and Agriculture Organization) and the OIE (World Organization for Animal Health), is working in this direction. The resurgence and emergence of infectious diseases, of which the Covid-19 crisis was the culmination, have been the focus of this initiative since the early 2000s. The principle is simple: protecting human health involves protecting the health of animals and entire ecosystems, considering that almost two-thirds of infectious diseases that affect humans are zoonoses, in other words, diseases of animal origin, and that there is probably a link between the degradation of biodiversity and the emergence of these new zoonoses.

---

13 Available at: https://www.fondationbiodiversite.fr/en/biodiversity-challenges/biodiversity-and-health/.

The One Health concept is aimed at everyone and advocates a global approach. In France, for example, ANSES (*Agence nationale pour la sécurité sanitaire de l'alimentation, de l'environnement et du travail*, the French National Agency for Food, Environmental and Occupational Health & Safety) advocates this approach in its numerous fields of intervention and encourages work in many areas, such as the spread of vectors, the impacts of climate change on workers' health and antibiotic resistance.

The tourism sector could also contribute to this concept through its activities, particularly in natural and protected areas that are promoted for tourism. However, the One Health initiative does not, for the moment, appear in the various bodies working to promote sustainable tourism.

4.2.2. *Example: the impact of cruise tourism*

In an article published in 2011, Klein questions the challenges of cruise tourism through the prism of responsible and sustainable tourism. He identifies three main issues related to this activity.

Environmental issues related to environmental disruption caused by engines and their drag, the question of ballast discharges, wastewater treatment (more than 400 liters per day per passenger) and fuel and oil effluents; air pollution from engines; solid waste management, requiring treatment. These nuisances have an indirect impact on the health of local populations.

Economic issues, in that the benefits derived from the activities offered during the ports of call are not always (or are rarely) redistributed equitably in the local economies. Moreover, welcoming cruise ships requires significant investments in infrastructures.

Socio-cultural issues that impact the quality of life of local populations. The sudden arrival of a large number of tourists disembarking at a port of call can cause major problems and totally saturate the space. Therefore, the disadvantages of tourism far outweigh its advantages. The United Nations Committee on Tourism and Sustainability notes that when the capacity of a port of call is exceeded, the general cost of living is affected, and temporary overcrowding and noise pollution are harmful to local populations and can lead to the rejection of tourism, which is what happened in the Florida Keys archipelago and led to demonstrations for a reduction in the number of tourists disembarking.

However, the recent SARS-CoV-2 (or Covid-19) global pandemic has shed new light on the relationship between health and cruising as a form of tourism, through the now emblematic case of the Diamond Princess. The luxury liner departed from

Hong Kong on January 13, 2020, with 2,666 passengers and 1,045 crew members on board. Twelve days later, an 80-year-old passenger disembarked with worrisome symptoms and a fever. A week later, the results were in: the culprit was the coronavirus. Then, on February 3, 2020, while the global pandemic was still in its infancy, the ship entered the port of Yokohama, Japan, where the Japanese authorities imposed a 14-day quarantine. The coronavirus that had begun to circulate in isolation on board the liner eventually contaminated 619 passengers and claimed the lives of seven of them. The story is eloquent in many ways: first, the octogenarian considered to be patient zero, although in poor health, did not go to the ship's medical center while traveling and continued to rub shoulders with the other passengers, thus spreading the disease by contagion. This then required a search and identification of all the people who had close contact with them. This proved to be insufficient and the number of cases grew rapidly to 135 after a week of quarantine, despite the confinement of passengers to their cabins. After 14 days, some of the passengers who tested negative could disembark, while the others remained under surveillance for some time. The lack of preparation for the risk of propagation of an infectious disease on board ship and the absence of prevention that led patient zero to take no measures to avoid contaminating the other passengers are revealing of the fact that health is relatively overlooked by the tourism sector and ultimately only triggers reflection and action in response to crises.

Looking at the longer term, cruises were shut down from March to September 2020, causing, according to a Cruise Line International Association report, a loss of €64 billion and 518,000 jobs for the industry worldwide[14] (and, according to an article in the newspaper *Ouest France*, many companies had not resumed operations by mid-February 2021). The cruise industry is trying to adapt by opting for rigorous health protocols (tests on boarding, wearing of masks and social distancing on board, reinforced medical logistics on ships and also strict protocols during stopovers). The American health authorities now require cruise ships to have a laboratory on board for passenger testing.

The Covid-19 health crisis will therefore have had a lasting impact on this sector and will have instilled a health dimension into its operating standards. However, there is no guarantee that health-related concerns will go beyond the limits of crisis management to join the more global concerns of sustainable tourism.

4.2.3. *Social environment*

The processes of land-use planning and urbanization that often accompany tourism development can, if not controlled and regulated, generate phenomena

14 Available at: https://cruising.org/-/media/research-updates/research/2021-state-of-the-cruise-industry_optimized.ashx.

of impoverishment and gentrification with a strong impact on local societies (Cocola-Gant 2018). Impoverishment will affect neighborhoods where tourism workers and, especially, seasonal workers live, relegated to the margins of the tourism-enhanced space. Conversely, gentrification is taking place in those valued areas where land prices tend to rise sharply, which selects inhabitants according to their financial capacities and once again pushes the less well-off to the margins. In terms of health, these processes are not neutral. In simple (and perhaps simplistic, according to (Bourdin 2008)) terms, gentrification describes a process whereby the wealthy classes reinvest in spaces that are abandoned in varying degrees and "drive out" the poorest. There are two aspects to this phenomenon when applied to tourist areas. On the one hand, it is accompanied by the renovation of certain neighborhoods, the development of an attractive cultural life and services (including healthcare services). On the other hand, it can increase inequality and lead to areas favoring a more gentrified clientele, which, in terms of health, translates into a two-tier system. Research in the field of health has not shown any direct or systematic causal link between gentrification and health issues, but according to Smith et al. (2020), the evidence accumulated in a literature review on gentrification in the United States shows a negative impact on the health of two categories of population: African Americans and those at the lowest income levels. The causes seem to be the difficulty that these populations have in maintaining their social network in the face of urban changes and their residential mobility, and yet social networks are identified in social epidemiology as a major determinant of health.

Transposed to tourism, these observations suggest that fragile population groups may be exposed to negative health effects in areas affected by gentrification. A study conducted in the Gòtic district of Barcelona supports this view (Sánchez-Ledesma et al. 2020). The authors identify seven categories that form a framework for understanding the links between tourism-related gentrification and population health: (1) the decline of social networks, (2) a loss of identity, (3) environmental changes, (4) pollution, (5) changes in available services, (6) real estate speculation and evictions and (7) resident activism. In other words, it is jointly the modification of the built environment, the social environment and the associated psychological factors that negatively impact health, both physical and mental (resulting in respiratory diseases, poor nutritional habits, sleep disorders, stress, anxiety and even depression). Resident activism was seen to absorb the negative health effects of living in a tourist area.

Gentrification is just one example of the impact of tourism on the social environment with consequences on health. In a recent article (Fleuret and Marie-dit-Chirot 2020), we highlighted the psychological suffering of tourism workers on the Riviera Maya in Mexico, linked, in particular, to the absence of solid social networks in a space that is populated mainly by migrants from various states around the country, coupled with a lack of psychiatric care. This suffering was accentuated by the difficult working conditions and the meeting of two worlds, one coming to recharge its batteries on vacation and the other working hard in their service.

4.3. Social health impacts

The impact of tourism on the social environment of vacation destinations has both direct and indirect repercussions on the health of local populations. These impacts can be understood in different ways: by population groups (such as workers in the tourism sector), by type of impact (such as alterations in traditional ways of life) or by a microgeography of tourism pressure in a location (e.g. by seeking to link the notion of carrying capacity with health).

4.3.1. *Occupational health*

Although tourism is one of the biggest economic sectors in terms of job and business creation, it is not particularly impacted by technology and automation (Baum et al. 2016) and therefore relies heavily on the labor of a heterogeneous workforce. Tourism occupations are very diverse, but one trend stands out overall:

> Jobs in tourism are primarily precarious due to the overrepresentation of atypical employment contracts structured around flexibility and mobility, such as those for seasonal and temporary workers, but also used for the huge number of subcontractors (hotel cleaning and laundry, janitorial services, and so on). New forms of flexible employment, mostly contract work, have also developed as a result of the so-called collaborative economy (such as for drivers and guides). To this must be added the significant use of casual work. The weakness and above all the variability and uncertainty of remuneration appear to be at the heart of the precariousness of tourism workers (Demeyère 2020).

Little is known on the subject of working conditions in the tourism sector, and a fortiori the health issues, according to Baum et al. (2016). According to Demeyère (2020), this is a "neglected aspect of the social responsibility of tourism-related organizations". In Spain, the work of Cañada (2015–2018) on hotel chambermaids has revealed to the general public the harsh working conditions of those who call themselves *kellys* (short for "las *que li*mpian los hotels", those who clean hotels). The results of this study show that recent developments in hotel management (particularly following the financial crisis of 2008) have resulted in: a deterioration of working conditions involving, simultaneously, a drop in pay levels and a devaluation of professional qualifications; an increase in the workload; irregular hours (whether relating to the duration of contracts or the predictability and regularity of schedules);

segmentation and division of tasks that puts the staff of the same hotel workforce in competition, rather than collaborating with each other; a decline in the capacity of workers to defend their interests; and, finally, a rise in health problems. Indeed, there are numerous health impacts from deteriorating working conditions which are directly linked to the way the sector operates, especially in its recent tendency to develop "low-cost" offerings to attract an ever-increasing number of customers who are still little aware of and little concerned about living a tourist experience that relies on the mistreatment of employees in the sector. Mistreatment is indeed the word used by Kokabi and NnoMan (2020) in an article reporting on the strike by chambermaids employed as subcontractors by the Accor group for the Ibis Batignolles hotel in Paris. For these chambermaids, by resorting to subcontractors, hotel groups "get rid of the issue of work drudgery at the same time. The job of a chambermaid is very hard work and the day one of them is partially unfit, the hotelier does not give a damn and just tells the subcontractor to get on with it (sic)". Paid by the number of rooms cleaned whereas the hotel employees are paid by the hour, subcontractors do not benefit from the same social protection and in order to hope for a barely correct level of remuneration, they must adopt a hellish pace. "They have to clean three and a half rooms per hour, which is simply impossible. To reach their targets, they work overtime, which is not taken into account and unpaid. They work themselves to death: many of them get sick and suffer with tendonitis, back pain or carpal tunnel syndrome."

Occupational illnesses in the tourism sector are just as varied as the professions. Principally among them are musculoskeletal disorders linked to repetitive tasks and load carrying, disorders linked to chronic fatigue generated by excessive working hours and a whole range of psychological disorders, linked to stress and insecurity in particular. This is a very competitive work environment, marked by excessive hours and workloads: frequently, employees have only one day off per week, with working days ranging from 8 to 12 hours. Life in these conditions is almost exclusively punctuated by work, and many of the employees we met said that they do not even have time to wash their clothes or take care of their children, let alone have time for themselves. For example, a hotel employee we met in Tulum, Mexico, explained that she works from dawn to dusk six days a week and that, due to traffic problems, it can take her up to an hour to get to work and the same amount of time to return. When she arrives home, she just wants to take a bath and sleep. She is not hungry and so either does not eat or she eats nachos or some other junk food. When she has a day off, she sleeps and does nothing else. Have some leisure time? She has not even thought about it. She would like to change her job, to grow, but even thinking about what she could do seems insurmountable to her as she does not have the head space for it.

The issue of psychological suffering among workers in the tourism sector is further aggravated by certain characteristics. This is a sector where seasonality is strong, which leads to a very intense work rhythm concentrated over a few months, followed by periods of inactivity that are not always covered by employment insurance. For example, in Mexico's Yucatán Peninsula, September is the off-season and tourism companies have fewer jobs to offer, which means that many workers find themselves unemployed. The month of September (*Septiembre* in Spanish) has been renamed *Septi-hambre* (*hambre* meaning hunger).

While Quintana Roo is known internationally for its sandy beaches and resorts that are popular with tourists, the state has one of the highest suicide rates in the country at 8.2 cases per 100,000 inhabitants in 2017, which puts it in fifth place among the 32 Mexican states, and significantly above the national average of 5.2 cases per 100,000 inhabitants in the same year (INEGI 2017). Quintana Roo registers similar trends for other pathologies, such as anxiety disorders, which affect 14% of the working population, compared with 7% nationally, and even alcoholism (Escobar et al. 2018).

The attractiveness of jobs in tourism and the location of destinations mean that many workers in the sector have experienced one or more migrations, and their life trajectories are complex and marked by uprooting, which weakens the social supports that are essential for health during hard times. If we look again at the situation in the Yucatán Peninsula, a tourist conurbation such as the Riviera Maya, that stretches from Cancún to Tulum, has grown from almost zero population in the mid-1970s to more than 1.5 million inhabitants, mainly from neighboring Mexican states (In 2010, 53% of the resident population declared that they had been born in another region of Mexico). Displacement, loneliness and difficulties in adapting to local society are all factors in psychological unease and suffering, even in the context of internal migrations within the same country (Luna Garcia 2019).

Health and especially mental health infrastructures are lagging behind this rapid population growth. Quintana Roo is in fact a poor relation of the Mexican mental health system and despite the glaring problem of increased psychological suffering in the tourist sector, it is one of the seven states out of 32 without a single psychiatric hospital. The situation is also critical in terms of the number of psychiatrists: the state had only 19 in 2016, a rate of 1.27 per 100,000 inhabitants, while the national average in the same year was 3.68 per 100,000 inhabitants (Heinze et al. 2016). In Playa del Carmen, a city of over 200,000 inhabitants, there were only four. This problem of deficiency in the mental health sector is widespread in many international tourist destinations (Figure 4.6).

Access to medication is another glaring problem. Faced with this situation, civil society is reacting and the associative sector has taken the initiative to develop services – especially for suicide prevention – gradually leading the public authorities to take note of the problem: recently, a mental health center was opened in Playa del Carmen with the support of the municipality, and the state of Quintana Roo published a mental health bill in 2020. Unfortunately, the Covid-19 crisis occurred and has impacted the tourism sector and dried up financial sources. Therefore, there is total uncertainty today about the outcome of these developments.

The problem of health at work in the tourism sector is not inexorable: solutions exist and employers can play a very positive role. For example, some hotels offer a "health training" program that includes physical activity, nutritional advice and support for stress and anxiety management, as well as corporate medical insurance that is far more beneficial than what employees might have access to within poor healthcare systems.

Another initiative worth mentioning is the European OiRA (Online interactive Risk Assessment) project, which offers online tools enabling micro and small enterprises to assess the occupational safety and health (OSH) risks in their activity and to improve working conditions and health of their employees. OiRA's tools are sector-specific: for tourism, there is a tool dedicated to the hotel and restaurant industry and another dedicated to sports and leisure activities[15].

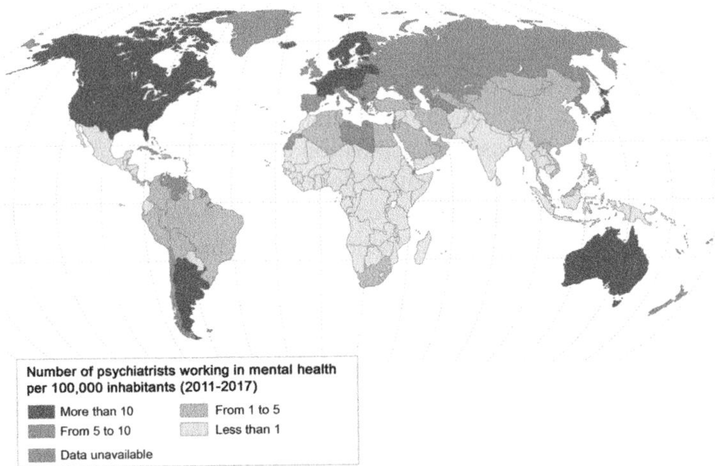

Figure 4.6. *Psychiatrists around the world (source: World Health Organization, 2011–2017; background map: FNSP. Sciences Po - Cartography workshop CC BY 4.0; design and production: S. Fleuret, A. Lepetit, UMR 6590 ESO)*

Solutions do exist, but they will only be effective if the tourism sector becomes aware of the issues related to occupational health, which will probably require an increase in research in this field. Baum et al. (2016) demonstrated, based on a broad review of the literature, that working conditions in the tourism and hotel sectors are a largely neglected subject.

15 Available at: https://oiraproject.eu/en/oira-tools.

4.3.2. *Changing lifestyles: thoughts on food*

Tourism brings together societies with very different practices and lifestyles, and tourists often bring diseases and other health problems to indigenous peoples. However, although tourists are familiar with these problems and know how to deal with them, this is not always the case for the populations at their destination (Richter 2003).

The question of food is a good example of this problem. Tourism has an impact on food lifestyles in at least two ways: the first is an impact on prices, which tend to be driven up by this market of potential customers with high purchasing power and by the demand generated by the hotel and restaurant sector; the second is through copying or diffusion of western standards that can result in interculturation (a kind of food syncretism) or acculturation (more radical transformation of habits).

The changes in dietary practices are resulting in a greater intake of proteins through meat, lipids, sugars and salt through processed food products. The corollaries of these changes are an increase in obesity and the emergence of cardiovascular diseases in indigenous societies.

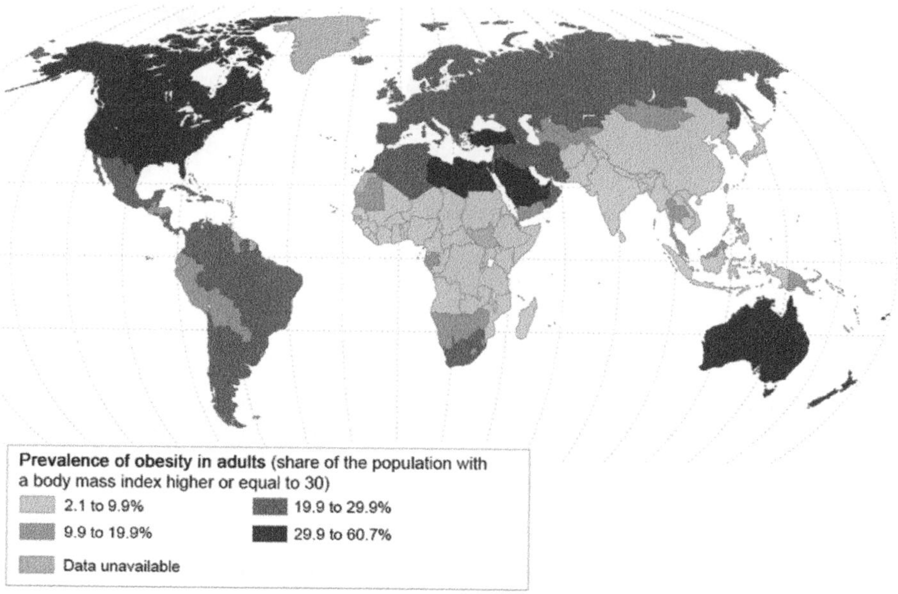

Figure 4.7. *Variations in body mass index around the world (source: World Health Organization, The Global Health Observatory, NCD risk factors: Overweight/Obesity, 2016; background map: FNSP Sciences Po – Cartography workshop CC BY 4.0; design and production: S. Fleuret, A. Lepetit, UMR 6590 ESO)*

Tourism is therefore actively participating in the spread of fast food, the junk food model, and thus in the global spread of the obesity epidemic (Théry and Caron 2019), which now affects the Asian and African continents (Figures 4.7 and 4.8). To date, there is no obesity mapping focused and adjusted on major tourist destinations, because the data analyzed in the main studies are national (Popkin and Gordon-Larsen 2004), but localized case studies suggest that tourism has an impact. For example, in Bali, Suastika et al. (2011) conducted a study on the prevalence of obesity and diabetes in a panel of municipalities on the island, and it is clear that the localities of Legian and Ubud, the two highly tourist cities in the study, have obesity rates significantly higher than the national average of 35% (61.2% and 70.1%, respectively).

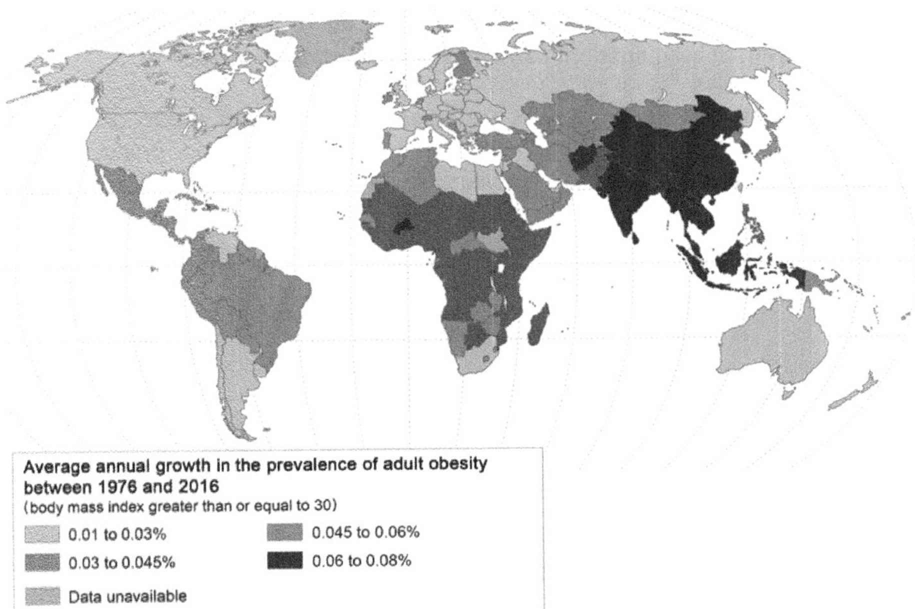

Figure 4.8. *Variations in the prevalence of obesity worldwide (source: World Health Organization, The Global Health Observatory, NCD risk factors: Overweight/Obesity, 2016. Map background: FNSP Sciences Po – Cartography workshop CC BY 4.0; design and production: S. Fleuret, A. Lepetit, UMR 6590 ESO)*

Our observations in the tourist region of the Riviera Maya, Mexico, point in this direction. More than 60% of the food consumed in Quintana Roo is imported, fast food is abundant and it is easier to buy sugared or sweetened sodas than water.

However, some countries have a dietary tradition based on nutritionally virtuous regimes that can be an argument for attracting tourists. The Cretan diet, the principles of which are based on limiting saturated fats in food, has acquired a worldwide reputation. It is, in fact, a diet that is widespread throughout the Mediterranean region and many tourism operators have understood that there was a good opportunity to offer stays combining nutritherapy and physical activity, one example being a lodge in the Agadir hinterland, owned by a nutritionist doctor, which offers stays that combine a program to rebalance the diet with hikes in the coastal foothills of the High Atlas. Thus, contrary to the global trend of "macdonaldization", tourism can contribute to the propagation of practices aimed at good or healthy eating: the search for healthy, organic food, balanced dishes, reduction of meat consumption and so on. Vegetarian and even vegan restaurants are on the increase, making it possible to eat well-balanced meals in restaurants during a trip and meeting a strong demand[16]. This "healthy" trend has been accompanied by physical and well-being activities such as stretching sessions on the beach, yoga or various sports that take place in public spaces. Here again, local populations are impacted by what they see and by these practices that some will adopt by copying, but this time in a virtuous circle: as much as the introduction of junk food has led them to adopt bad practices to their detriment, so good practices can also be copied. Unfortunately, these processes are very socially unequal: the poorest adopt junk food (which is cheap and therefore accessible) and only the wealthy classes convert to organic food and have free time for sports on the beach.

More generally, for the tourism sector as a whole, we can note in this field other positive impacts imported with the tourists: the rise in sanitary standards, increases in hygiene and the possibility of finding products which did not previously exist in certain destinations (such as feminine hygiene products). This is accompanied by a slow but sure evolution of mentalities. For example, issues related to sexual health and the generalization of prevention messages on contraception are having a positive effect on family planning.

4.3.3. *Tourist carrying capacity and health issues*

According to Stock et al. (2003), carrying capacity is the number of visitors that a tourist site can accept without threatening a protected area (whether natural or cultural). This definition corresponds to that of the World Tourism Organization, which poses the problem in terms of potential damage to resources. This notion is discussed and criticized because of the difficulty of "simultaneously considering physical and ecological, social and economic, psychological, anthropological and cultural parameters..." (Cazes 1992). Stock et al. refer to the "impossible measurement of carrying capacity". However, if we go beyond the understanding of

16 Of course, there is also a part of greenwashing coming from some big restaurant chains to surf on this wave.

a tourist place seen as a resource (implying economic development through tourism) and if we integrate into the picture the degradations to the environment and the harmful impacts on biodiversity and human health, this notion cannot be dismissed out of hand, even if it is problematic. It is necessary to develop new investigations on this subject by including the environment and health. This takes place at different levels, and it is likely that tourism studies would benefit from being inspired by multilevel health analysis methods, which could provide solutions to the difficulties raised by G. Cazes.

A case in point, reported at the 2019 18th International Medical Geography Symposium in Queenstown, New Zealand, provides an excellent example of pressure from overcrowding through tourism.

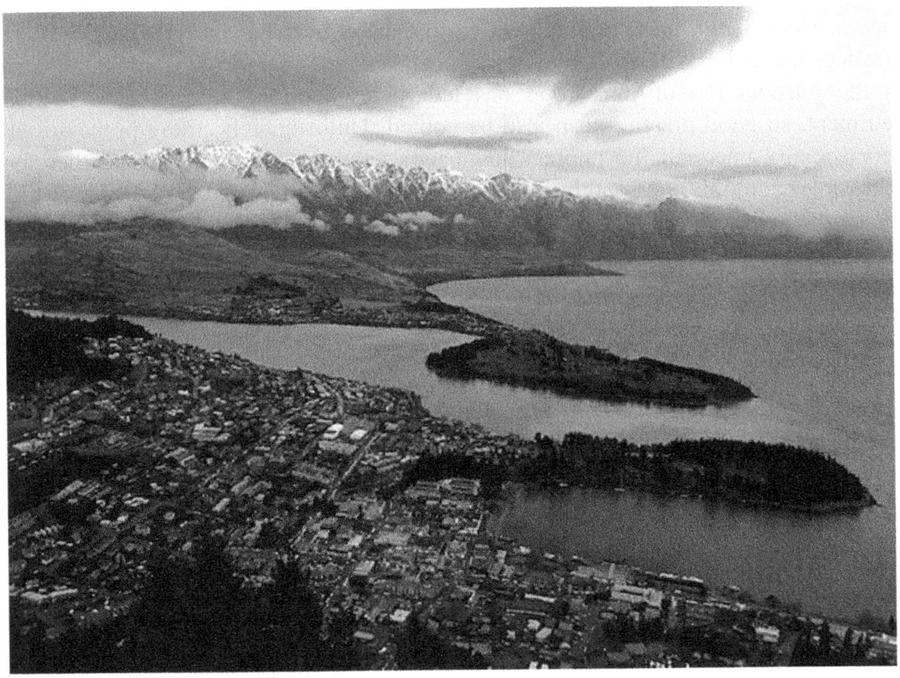

Figure 4.9. *Queenstown: the city seen from the top of the cable car above it (photo: S. Fleuret 2019)*

Queenstown is a city in the south of New Zealand with many tourist attractions: several ski resorts nearby, mountain tourism activities, the landscape in which P. Jackson's film "The Lord of the Rings", based on Tolkien's book, was shot, a beautiful lake and so on.

This small city of 15,000 inhabitants welcomes 3 million tourists per year and, according to its local elected officials, is therefore permanently faced with an overpopulation that must be fed and which generates nuisances and pollution (particularly road traffic that causes congestion that is worthy of a metropolis). It was during an environmental and health crisis that a diagnosis was made and led to thinking about mechanisms for regulating tourist pressure in order to preserve not only the resource but also the health of the population and of visitors. This crisis occurred in connection with agriculture, relating to the increase in the breeding of livestock in order to satisfy the growing needs of tourists. The development of livestock farming has resulted in an increase in environmental pressure: the manure produced has infiltrated the groundwater and, with it, the *Escherichia coli* bacteria. The magnitude of the phenomenon eventually made the water undrinkable and required that a lake be closed to swimming for a period of several weeks, handicapping tourist activity. This event acted as a wake-up call and other indirect consequences of tourism overload on quality of life and health began to be studied in a systemic approach. Thus, another indirect effect has been identified, starting with the increase in the price of land caused by the dynamics of buying second homes. The local population, no longer able to buy real estate near the center, must move away from the city to find affordable land and therefore commute by car to and from work. This results in a change in their lifestyle, stress, fatigue and negative impacts on health. In addition, the deterioration of housing conditions for those who are not able to buy their own home also has consequences and the first to be affected are the poorest. Here again, certain manifestations linked to degraded housing translate into health symptoms (such as an increase in respiratory diseases).

Many other direct and indirect impacts could be listed around this case (pressure on the capacity of healthcare facilities, for instance). What should be retained from this established link between tourism overload and environmental and health impacts is the need for regulatory mechanisms. For the local authorities in Queenstown, taxation (tourist taxes, for example) can be used for this. We will see in the next chapter that diagnostic tools are beginning to be developed and allow health impact assessments (HIAs) to accompany development projects for tourist destinations and attractions.

5

Health, Ignored in Tourism Development? A Neglected Asset?

The observation that health is one of the poor relations of tourism studies is a common theme running through the aspects mentioned in the previous four chapters, a neglected issue that only becomes a concern when crises (whether health or environmental) occur. The issues related to health in tourism development are not well known and are largely underestimated. The health impacts and consequences of the growth of this sector and its ever-increasing internationalization are also largely neglected, or even ignored. Yet, we may well ask ourselves if health would not be such a neglected asset, and would be a high-potential tourist segment, if the players in the sector were to take up the issue. More broadly, we may wonder whether, in a post-Covid context, the issues linking tourism and health might not constitute an opportunity to change the paradigm and finally integrate the "health" dimension into the development of territories through tourism.

5.1. Health and wellness as a tourist segment

In Chapter 3, we discussed medical tourism, but this is part of a broader field that we call health and wellness tourism. Interviewed by Stettler for a Swiss magazine on gastronomy and hospitality (2018), in an article that invites hoteliers to consider health tourism as a real opportunity and to position themselves clearly, researcher M. Smith of the University of Budapest lists the factors that influence health tourism (Box 5.1). The list is long and varied: it includes biomedical motivations (related to the body and its appearance, to its "maintenance" in the face of the effects of age or the modern pace of life) and medical-psychological motivations (such as stress management, self-esteem and the treatment of addictions), as well as motivations that refer to a holistic vision of health and well-being (the search for happiness, self-esteem and spirituality). A distrust of allopathic medicine is also a motivating factor for health tourism based on alternative care. Finally, life situations, such as loneliness or the feeling of being locked into a life that is too complicated, can give rise to a desire to escape for the time of a tourist stay, the main purpose of which will be self-care.

– Mental and physical exhaustion.

– Wishing to be healthier.

– Stress due to work and the pace of life.

– Wishing to be happier.

– Lack of trust in traditional medical care.

– Desire for active aging over the long term.

– Loneliness.

– Needing to develop self-esteem.

– Obsession with self-image.

– Desiring to be thinner, more beautiful and to look younger.

– Desire for spirituality.

– Need for rehabilitation.

– Dependence on new technologies.

– Wishing to live a simpler life.

Box 5.1. *Factors influencing health tourism (source: Budapest Metropolitan University/Gastrojournal.ch)*

Hoteliers, but more broadly the whole tourism industry, have, in health tourism, a segment to develop, provided that they position themselves beyond the restrictive approach of medical tourism, which, we recall, is defined by the aim of medical tourists, which is to cure an illness or an ailment and/or to access a better quality of care or different treatments to those they could find at home. This tourism involves medical approaches and therefore health professionals.

However, the health tourism segment includes two other types of offer: wellness (or well-being), which does not target the sick, but individuals who are looking to do themselves good, to take care of themselves, for example, with massages. Then, at the midpoint between medical and wellness tourism, we find medical wellness, which proposes stays including activities that explicitly aim to maintain or improve personal health and well-being (nutrition cures, anti-aging, etc.). These therapeutic stays may include a medical dimension, but this is not always the case, rather more of a tourist practice focused on generally improving the quality of life.

The hotel services and activities that mark the stay will differ according to the chosen location, and, depending on the case, tourism operators can either develop their offer completely independently or join forces with a health partner, a doctor or a private clinic; we will return to this later. The idea is to include a health offer as part of a package that combines time for self-care (such as yoga courses) with excursions, the possibility of participating in sports, shopping or even ecotourism activities or simply hiking or lounging on the beach.

This form of tourism, linked to local health and wellness infrastructures, has great potential. According to a study conducted across 50 destinations (Smith and Puczkó 2015), 43% of people who visit these facilities are actually tourists.

5.1.1. *Health benefits of travel and tourism*

Travel and tourism have beneficial impacts on health, as do all leisure activities, the positive impact of which has been measured more frequently in scientific studies. Pressman et al. (2009) showed, for example, that participation in recreational activities was associated with positive health effects measured through the following indicators: blood pressure, cortisol (cholesterol) levels, waist circumference and body mass index, as well as a better self-perception of physical abilities. Bessy (1991) referred to this intersection between health and sport as “fitness tourism”, and several medical studies on cohorts have sought to demonstrate the benefits of the so-called “active” travel (Saunders et al. 2013), that is, requiring physical effort (walking, cycling, rowing, etc.). These studies concluded that benefits exist, notably for obesity and diabetes as well as on child health, but that it is very complicated to demonstrate them medically. This is probably one of the reasons why health is struggling to become a dynamic in tourism.

Generally, according to Borins (2000), “there is something therapeutic about getting away from everyday routines and being exposed to different environments”, but, as is often the case in health studies, it is through a negative effect (such as in photography) that we can provide some evidence to support this intuition. For example, Eaker and Castelli (1992) measured the negative effects of not taking a vacation on a cohort of women followed for 20 years. Those who took few or no vacations were significantly more likely to suffer a myocardial infarction. The risk ratio doubled between women who reported not taking a vacation for six or more years and those who reported going away either every year or several times a year. Despite a certain lack of research on physical health, several studies reported by

Borins (2000) or Chen and Petrick[1] (2013), among others, have shown an impact of taking a vacation on life expectancy, on mental health (particularly depression or burn-out) and on numerous physiological indicators, such as: reduction in stress hormone levels, better sleep and lower blood pressure. These health effects diminish over time following a return from vacation, which forms an argument for regularly renewing these periods of rest and travel (without necessarily having to travel far away). These findings suggest that vacation stays, even though they have a cost, have many benefits, and it would probably be pertinent to calculate whether they would not largely outweigh the initial costs when converted into health and therapy costs following a lack of vacation.

Yet, surprisingly, health is almost absent from the commercial argument in tourism, with the notable exception of its holistic denomination: well-being. Is it the relative absence of medical studies on this subject that is to blame, or, conversely, is it the lack of enthusiasm within the tourism sector for these issues that keeps research levels low?

5.1.2. *Health, well-being and tourist attractiveness*

Several studies have focused on the benefits of tourism on well-being (Proulx 2005; Smith and Puczkó 2008; Smith and Diekman 2017). Other studies (Sharpley 2014) have also focused on the impacts of tourism on the well-being of residents in destinations (this was discussed in Chapter 4). Much could be said about definitions of well-being that refer to both subjective and objective dimensions and raise measurement issues, which are all the more complex if we link them to health and if we wish to approach them from a territorial perspective (Fleuret and Atkinson 2007). In a particularly interesting text published in 2005 in the journal *Teoros*, Proulx, having identified various psychosociological (relaxation, entertainment and development), social (socialization, self-affirmation and personal belonging) and therapeutic functions of leisure, attributes "several personal and social benefits (that promote the health of families, neighborhoods and interest groups)" to these functions. According to Smith and Diekmann (2017), tourism is a way to satisfy certain desires (which refers to Maslow's 1954 work on the hierarchy of needs leading to well-being). For example, a trip is an opportunity to satisfy, even temporarily, a desire for change, even if, ultimately, the tourist experience is more or less partially idealized. For these authors, the well-being that the tourist experience can provide is both hedonistic (satisfaction of pleasures) and eudemonic (reinforcement of the feeling of accomplishment). However, as we have already seen, these two dimensions can come into conflict when, for example, the development of

1 In their review of the literature on the beneficial impacts of travel on health, these authors identified only 98 studies that actually fell within the scope of the analysis, which is very few.

low-cost tourism is based on altering the living and working conditions of employees in the sector.

In scientific literature, some forms of tourism are shown to be better linked to physical and mental well-being. This is the case, for example, with nature and climate tourism, including, for example, the field of research known as "blue spaces" research, in which different authors (Kruizinga 2016; Mc Namara et al. 2020) have studied the positive effects of visiting maritime spaces and practicing activities such as swimming. Other works have produced similar observations on visiting lakes (Konu et al. 2010), and we are now coming back to one of the foundations of tourism, which led to the development of thermalism and spas and which are now explicitly associated with wellness to argue the case for their attractiveness; indeed, several authors have also pointed out that spas are now selling "well-being" (Boiville 2005; Pépi et al. 2005). Sicsic (2018) also points out the risks of this trend:

> Tourism operators have always focused on selling pleasure based on the aesthetics of landscapes, the environment, nature, heritage, hospitality and leisure activities. However, today, they not only seek to sell relaxation and the physical sensations of well-being, but the most complex emotional state that exists; and often at astronomical prices. [...] A real economy has emerged that is bringing in tens of billions of dollars.

Referring to the book *Happycratie. Comment l'industrie du bonheur a pris le contrôle de nos vies* (its English title is *Manufacturing Happy Citizens: How the Science and Industry of Happiness Controls our Lives*), Sicsic reflects on whether the tourism sector, through some of its offerings, "realizes that it contributes to tyrannizing the individual by imposing a plethora of 'goods' intended to rectify his psychic weaknesses and overcome them in order to attain bliss". The question is worth asking, especially since it leads by extension to questions around the definition of well-being and the qualification of personnel (can one be qualified to provide well-being?).

In any event, the link between tourism and well-being is now well established, at least in the marketing and discourse, through combinations of activities carried out during a stay, the nature of which can promote self-fulfillment or self-realization, for instance. Smith and Diekmann (2008) cite, by way of illustration, packages that combine purely hedonistic tourist experiences with eudemonic, "meaningful" activities, volunteer work or cultural experiences. Based on their analyses, these authors propose an image of tourism that integrates the dimensions of well-being and is thus positioned at the intersection between pleasure, self-realization and altruism (Figure 5.1). The challenge for tourism operators is to be able to produce an offer that brings these three dimensions together, which is not an easy task as they vary so much according to individual subjectivity. This is, in fact, the same question as that posed by Hartwell et al. (2012) in the title of their article *Tourism engaging with the public health agenda: Can we promote wellville as a destination of choice?* This question amounts to imagining a strategy for tourism operators to promote the physical and mental well-being of both tourists and populations in destinations.

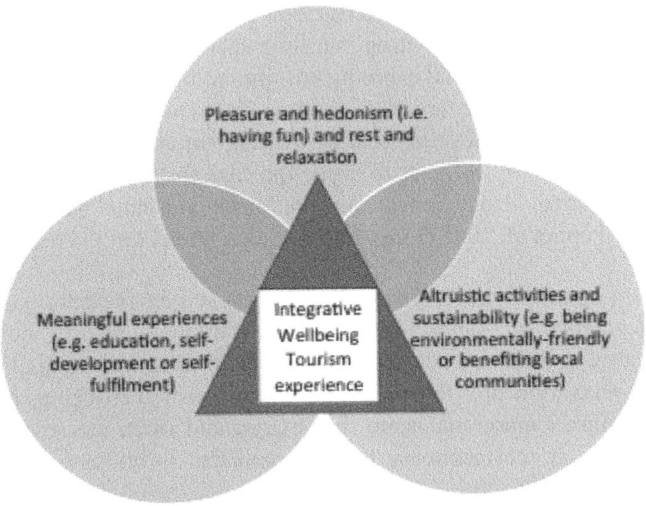

Figure 5.1. *Integrative well-being tourism experience according to Smith and Diekmann (2017). For a color version of all the figures in this chapter, see: www.iste.co.uk/fleuret/tourism.zip*

According to Hartwell et al., tourism does not exist in a vacuum and can only function if it shares, cooperates and has an effective dialogue with other sectors of society, while ensuring that it does not compromise the destination in terms of environmental, social and cultural integrity. This interface requires further study of the benefits of integration from a product, destination and environmental perspective and is discussed further below (section 5.4). With this premise in mind, the authors examine the situation in the United Kingdom, where a move to decentralize the healthcare system is transferring a certain number of competences locally, which appears to be an opportunity to create a common local culture between sectors of activity that were previously compartmentalized (tourism and health) and around a common ambition materialized by well-being:

> While both public health and tourism strategies can focus on promoting sustainability and reducing inequalities, evidence of such an approach is much stronger in the domain of public health. However,

> consistent with the values of sustainable tourism, these can be mapped on to a range of tourism policy determinants at the local level to aid a conceptualization of fusion between the two disciplines. Similarly, successful destination marketing may provide the economic impetus to transform local tourism products towards well-being; an approach that, for many destinations, can help counter the challenges posed by commodification [...] while, through its ability to influence policy and infrastructure, it may enhance healthy opportunities for residents.

Smith and Diekmann (2017) reach the same conclusion: "In terms of tourism development, it could be argued that destination planners need to adopt a utilitarian approach in order to ensure the well-being of the place and its people, as well as providing well-being enhancing experiences for tourists."

This ambition somewhat modifies "the traditional posture of the four S's (sea, sun, sand and sex) widespread in tourism marketing" and for Hobson and Dietrich (1995), it even questions "the responsibility of the actors to continue to base their strategies on these four S's". It is now a question of integrating the tourism economy into a set of non-medical determinants of health and not losing sight of the fact that the strategic choices made can have positive or harmful effects.

5.2. Synthesis of potentials

Once we consider the fact that health tourism is a neglected segment, the question arises: what are the potentials that should be developed? The following sections attempt to provide an answer in the form of a synthesis.

5.2.1. *Flagship products*

Flagship products stand out in the wellness and health tourism markets: thermalism, thalassotherapy, balneotherapy and spas. Recently, new complementary offers have emerged, all of which are riding on the back of the fashionable market of well-being, of "self-care". This is about taking care of your body through massages, or sports activities aimed at health wellness, or even through treatments often backed by a product identified as natural and regional. The offer is plethoric and eclectic: in Europe, for example, we can cite vinotherapy combined with wine tourism, which offers treatments based on wine derivatives (e.g. skin care with wine lees, which are reputed to be anti-oxidant). This offer is a way for wineries to diversify their tourism activity by distinguishing themselves from the classic bed and breakfast and farm tourism markets. A French brand, Caudalie, has particularly positioned itself within this segment and provides cosmetic and well-being products derived from the vine that are used in the tourism offer.

Many destinations seek to capitalize on their local production by emphasizing a relaxing or therapeutic use of these local products. This is the case, as discussed in a previous chapter, with the Sousse Massa region in Morocco (around Agadir) where massages using argan oil are offered to tourists. In the south of Morocco (and in some other Maghreb countries), there are those who seek to take advantage of the desert with sand therapy, which consists of being buried in hot sand to improve blood pressure, relieve certain joint pains and promote sweating and exfoliation. There, as elsewhere, this tourist offer around wellness treatments is developing and tends to take various forms (such as nutritherapy stays, meditation retreats and reflexology). This potential is being exploited by hoteliers (increasing numbers of whom are equipping themselves with spa relaxation areas), as well as by a range of local actors (such as masseurs on the beaches) and can be seen as an offer that allows for the renewal of the attractiveness of crisis-affected tourist areas, as the growth of this segment of activity was estimated at 7% per year in 2015[2].

The construction of a marketing strategy that integrates the health and well-being dimension therefore consists of suggesting to the tourist that, in addition to resting, they can recharge their batteries, eat well, take care of their body and mind and take care of themselves.

5.2.2. *An evolving clientele*

The evolution of clientele is the second parameter to be considered, and, in particular, population aging, which is accompanied by the development of a seniors offer that is not a replacement for, but is added to, the classic offer. This seniors market has the particularity of being stable, composed of a population that displays a propensity to travel and spend, including (or even intentionally) during the low season, which allows order books to be filled and flows to be smoothed out over the year. Older tourists tend to have longer stays (see section 3.4). According to Lesserre and Chevalier (2013), three-quarters of people aged 65 and over go on vacation each year, and, during 2011, one in two people aged 70 and over traveled at least once over a distance of more than 100 km (data based on the French population). This is also a clientele for whom health is important "given that as individuals age, they are generally subject to an increasing number of health-related problems, from vision and hearing problems to digestive, knee and hip problems and cardiovascular

2 According to the CEO of Opodo France interviewed in an article in the newspaper *20 minutes* on the occasion of the World Tourism Fair in Paris (https://www.20minutes.fr/societe/1808515-20160317-mondial-tourisme-raisons-succes-sejours-bien-etre).

disease" (Leroux 2010). However, analyses of the composition of this market do not identify health as a key segmentation factor (Lesserre and Chevalier, *op. cit.*), even though our field observations in two destinations (Agadir in Morocco and Saly in Senegal) have shown that many senior citizens make their tourist trips for health reasons, in particular to seek out a climate and a restful living environment that are more favorable to their health. In the scientific literature that associates it with tourism, health is more often considered in terms of the possible consequences of travel (Hunter-Jones 2003), or in terms of health problems that can limit the ability of seniors to travel, such as arthritis, diabetes and heart disease (Kabak 2004).

The seniors market is growing rapidly and is attracting the interest of players who see the "silver economy" as a highly lucrative field. However, it is necessary to make a very clear distinction between a tourism offer that includes health services, which is part of a gerontological approach as well as a social and health approach, and the silver economy, which is part of a commercial approach that excludes the most deprived and falls apart when dependency occurs. However, there are needs at this level: policies for maintaining people at home, as well as those for accommodating people in EHPADs (accommodation establishments for dependent elderly people) should include a tourism and leisure dimension and ensure that it is possible for elderly people to retain leisure activities at home and in the vicinity, as well as the ability to continue going on vacation. In institutions, leisure and entertainment activities exist, but several EHPAD managers are also thinking about how to send their residents on vacation for their individual benefit, which also has a secondary benefit for the institution as it allows them to be able to carry out maintenance, development or renovation work while residents are away. This type of stay is similar to the adapted stays already offered to disabled people. Finally, another potential is identified by Hunter Jones and Blackburn (2007): tourism that allows the elderly to travel together with their caregivers, who compensate for their disabilities all year round and are exhausted by this task, who also have a crying need for the respite time that tourism can provide. The travel agencies and tourism operators that we interviewed at several tourism trade shows (in London and Madrid in 2020) seem not to have yet taken the measure of this potential, even though an adapted travel offer is starting to emerge.

5.2.3. *Four facets of the same object*

Ultimately, health and wellness tourism and well-being is a segment that is still too neglected, and yet it could be developed in view of the four facets that it presents and which are all attractive arguments for tourists.

The first is physical health, for which the tourism offer responds to different self-care needs, particularly through physical activity, healthcare and nutrition.

The second is mental health, for which tourism also offers prospects for resourcing, work on emotions, relaxation or even sensory awakening.

The third facet is linked to spiritual health and can be seen in the offers of tourist stays with a spiritual background that is not necessarily linked to a religious dimension: increasing numbers of operators are offering meditative retreats, for example, or retreats focused on a practice that combines healthcare and spirituality, such as Ayurveda.

The fourth facet is that of social health, which translates into benefits related to relationships, living together, team spirit and cohesion (e.g. in the context of business trips and potentially linked to a wellness and health at work approach).

These facets are interrelated and can be taken into account in a variety of ways in order to build products or even tourist destinations more or less based on the image of benefits for health and well-being that the tourist could derive from their stay. One destination in particular has exploited this positioning, namely the island of Bali, which sells its destination "as a tropical paradise: the island of the Gods" (Michel 2011), and which simultaneously communicates sports activities (surfing), food, preserved and rejuvenating nature (despite the ecological disasters at play), culture and spirituality, and body care (massages), thus touching all facets of health within the tourism offer. Bali's unique positioning probably derives from the local culture, which is imbued with the "*Tri Hita Karana* philosophy – which consists of maintaining harmonious relationships between humans and gods, humans and nature, and humans among each other – which feeds into the daily rituals and practices of local life, and this across all aspects: religion, rituals, agriculture, cuisine, arts, hotels, business, and so on" (Michel 2011).

However, Bali is a special case and very few destinations have realized the potential of health tourism and touted it as such.

Will Covid-19 act as a wake-up call? It is too soon to tell at the time of writing, as the pandemic is not yet over. Nevertheless, it seems that lessons will be learned from the cataclysm that the health crisis has represented for tourism, which will have been strongly affected by travel restrictions and social distancing measures. For the time being, this is reflected in specific measures, such as the street washbasins installed in Bali (Figure 5.2) or the systematization of health safety labels (such as the Safe Travels or Preverisk Group accreditations) that can be seen on hotel websites and comparison sites such as Booking.com or Tripadvisor.

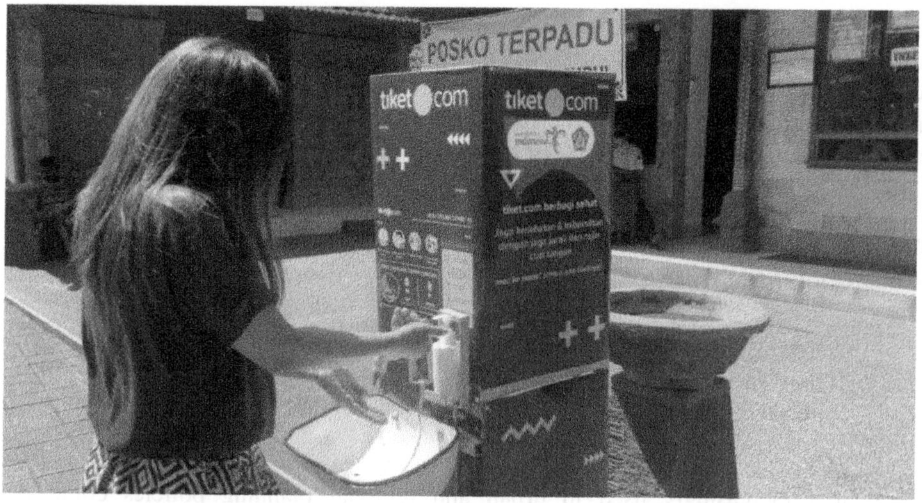

Figure 5.2. *Street handwash with disinfectant installed in Bali during the Covid-19 pandemic (source: The Jakarta Post, September 24, 2020). For a color version of all the figures in this chapter, see: www.iste.co.uk/fleuret/tourism.zip*

Some hotels have even completely modified their web pages (e.g. the Flamingo Hotel in Cancún). For the time being, the purpose of taking the health dimension into account in tourism is to reassure the traveler and is therefore a reaction to a crisis rather than an anticipation of the problem and even less a vision of health as an asset to develop or relaunch this activity.

5.3. What role for each category of actor?

Perhaps because it tends to be considered a sector of its own, health is often overlooked in urban and regional planning documents related to tourism. In work conducted in the Yucatán Peninsula (Fleuret and Jouault 2019), a review of Fonatur (Fondo Nacional de Fomento al Turismo) documents revealed the near-absence of health in the planning documents of the city of Cancún. In the 1970s, this tourist city literally sprang from the ground in a very structured planning process. Plans for its urban infrastructure, a modern electrical network, a water supply system, wide-paved avenues, an international airport and an impressive number of hotels were all laid down before being built, and the result of this planning is a city of 400,000 people with more than 140 hotels and over 26,000 rooms. And yet, in Fonatur's plans, only hygiene and sanitation were mentioned: not a word about healthcare facilities or public health infrastructure.

In order for health to be truly integrated into the discussions surrounding the development of tourism and the development of territories through tourism, several categories of actors present in the destination (and some in the sending territories) must concern themselves with the issue and take it on board. Three categories are affected: the actors of the territory, of health and of tourism.

5.3.1. *Territorial actors: assessing the health impacts of tourism development*

For the actors of the territory, one of the main challenges is integrating the health impacts of tourism development into the planning process, especially at the local level, in the same way as has been done in a long process regarding environmental impacts.

A tool increasingly used in urban and regional planning policies could be extended more systematically to the tourism sector: HIAs (Health Impact Assessments). According to the Gothenburg consensus paper (OMS/Centre européen pour les politiques de santé 1999), these are defined as "a combination of procedures, methods and tools by which a policy, program or project may be judged as to its potential effects on the health of a population, and the distribution of those effects within the population". According to this document, a health impact assessment is based on proven evidence about the predictable relationships of a policy, program or project on the health of the population. It must also include a democratic and participatory dimension, in other words, take into account the opinions, experiences and expectations of those who may be affected by the proposed policy, program or project. Finally, an HIA should serve to inform citizens, users of an infrastructure or beneficiaries of a development about the possible health effects of a policy, program or project. HIAs can be carried out upstream, downstream or during the course of a project and lead to proposals for adjustments or new options for increasing the positive effects and decreasing the negative aspects on health.

The approach is a recent one and still little known. Although it is gradually becoming established in the WHO Healthy Cities network, examples of HIAs conducted in the context of tourism projects are still rare.

In the Swiss Jura, for example, an HIA was carried out in the context of a project for a fossil discovery site. The objectives of this HIA were to evaluate the impacts (positive or negative) of this project on the health of local residents and tourists. The starting point for the assessment was the concern that the arrival of tourists in a rural area that is not very dense and not equipped to receive significant visitor numbers could have negative impacts on the environment and quality of life of the local inhabitants (such as transportation surges, air pollution and changes in the job market and working conditions). This HIA on the "Project to validate the dinosaur tracks in Courtedoux" made it possible to raise awareness among decision-makers of the public health issues involved in the project. The HIA approach is necessarily multidisciplinary but initiated by the actors of the territory.

Some countries are more advanced than others in this area. In Australia, HIAs are almost systematic. They are also widespread in the United Kingdom and Canada (particularly in Quebec). France is struggling to implement them, and they are very rare in the Southern Hemisphere.

One of the reasons which might explain why the health impacts of tourism have not been taken into account is the complexity of the phenomenon and the difficulties in measuring its direct and indirect, individual and population effects. In 1994, Lazzarotti wrote: "Nothing seems more difficult, therefore, than to untangle the jumble of chain reactions initiated by the irruption of tourism in any geographical environment." From there, he questioned the analysis methods and particularly the method based on cause and effect relationships, advocating a systemic approach widely used elsewhere in the field of public health. However, there is currently a serious lack of documented and supported studies dissecting the interactions, correlations and causalities between tourism and health. Yet, the stakes are high from the point of view of regional planning, which assumes an action of optimization of the use of space by the organization of the companies that practice it and through their activities (in this case, tourism). Indeed, is health not an essential indicator to be measured in order to be able to talk about optimization?

5.3.2. *Health actors: taking into account the fact of tourism*

While the territorial actors of tourism development and those of the tourism sector only very marginally integrate health issues into their prospective and operational reflections, the inverse is also true: the actors of health do not sufficiently take into account the tourism fact. One aspect of tourism is particularly revealing: seasonality. Surprisingly, seasonal variations in health supply and demand are not always integrated into health planning documents. Let us take the case of a large French tourist region: the *Schéma Régional d'Organisation Sanitaire* (SROS) of the Provence-Alpes-Côte d'Azur region (2012–2016) was particularly silent on this subject, even though the PACA region is one of the main summer tourist destinations in France, and this version of the SROS immediately followed the promulgation of the so-called HPST (*Hôpital, Patient, Santé Territoire* – hospital, patient and health territory) Act, which provided for regional health plans to be based on territorial diagnostics. By neglecting the impact of tourism, this document demonstrates that health is a relative unknown in health planning. However, seasonal variations in health needs are significant due to the number of tourists welcomed (31 million stays per year, a 60% increase in the population in summer) and the number of seasonal workers attracted (nearly 150,000). In this region, the challenges are not only in terms of problems of access to healthcare for the local population due to the increased demand by summer visitors (see section 4.1.1), but also in terms of the equitable distribution of services. The supply of services is concentrated on the coast (tourist and urbanized) to the detriment of a rural and neglected hinterland. Tourism also introduces specific problems and would require health planning to follow a methodology adapted to tourist areas and to the very nature of tourist activities. This is the case in mountain areas where sports with trauma risks are practiced, which will, for example, justify the establishment of a radiologist close to a ski resort. This is much less the case in coastal areas, and if we no longer look at the needs of tourists but at those of workers in the sector, the oversight is even more obvious, which caused C. Demeyère (2020) to say that health is a "neglected aspect of social responsibility" in the tourism sector. However, the responsibility does not lie entirely with the tourism sector, or just with the health sector, and each must make a move towards the other.

5.3.3. *Tourism stakeholders: linking tourism and health*

One of the main challenges for tourism actors in integrating health in their activity is their ability to build partnerships with the medical and healthcare world.

In the field of health tourism (taken in its broadest sense, from medical tourism to wellness tourism), we are witnessing the development of "clusters" that can be defined as sets of "interdependent companies (belonging to the health field as well as to tourism and leisure) working in the same sector and collaborating strategically to obtain common benefits" (Ramirez Karla et al. 2017). The objective of this approach is to jointly capture the windfall of health-related tourist spending. These clusters can take various forms, ranging from simple collaboration between operators in the two sectors to highly integrated "Medicity" models, as discussed in 2012 by Chasles using the example of Medanta, a medicity in Gurgaon, near Delhi (www.medenta.org). These medical complexes "combine state-of-the-art medicine with competitive prices, in an environment containing modern hospitals as well as hotel complexes, apartments and private companies". The main target of health tourism clusters is the medical tourist, the naming of which is open to criticism (see section 3.1) because this tourist ultimately barely benefits from the amenities of the destination, other than its healthcare facilities. The objective of the clusters is therefore, essentially, to coordinate tour operators, airport transfer companies, hotels and healthcare establishments. One area that is still largely underestimated and, yet, has great potential is that of accompanying family members, who could be offered activities or excursions, rather than remaining continuously at the bedside of the patient they are accompanying.

These clusters are still few and far between, and examples that include the non-medical branches of health tourism (whether it be the wellness offer in general or paramedical offers such as a cure, for example) are rare. However, when such examples do exist, it is the entire destination that becomes a form of cluster. In the principality of Andorra, the public body in charge of promoting tourism in the region (Andora Turisme) has created the Andorra Health Destination initiative (https://healthdestination.ad/fr), in which 15 partners come together to offer tourists a variety of experiences centered on well-being and health. This program brings together qualified professionals in these fields and promotes the fact that the care and treatments offered draw on the natural resources of the Andorran territory, a healthy environment of lakes, mountains and a high-quality climate. Among the experiences offered on the program's website, we find, in no particular order, stays for the treatment of chronic pain (3 or 4 days), two-day anti-stress escapades to combat burn-out, physiotherapy stays, anti-aging cures, yoga courses (from 3 to 5 days) and even thermal cures accompanied by Ayurveda therapy and so on.

In another example, the Auvergne-Rhône-Alpes region in France has created a telephone platform in partnership with health professionals, who are there to advise travelers so that they can choose a tailor-made stay that combines a tourism experience with well-being. This platform is 100% free and is called *Destination Santé et Bien-être* ("Destination Health and Wellness") (https://pro.auvergnerhone alpes-tourisme.com/destination-sante-et-bien-etre/). It is primarily intended for tourism professionals for whom it is a resource for communicating with future clients when they have a health-related question prior to a reservation.

The first, admittedly tentative, steps towards linking tourism actors with those of health and the territories have therefore been taken. Certain geographical areas appear to be taking the subject in hand, such as in Spain and more widely in the Spanish-speaking world, as evidenced by the existence of a pavilion reserved for the theme of tourism and health, entitled "Health Fitur", at the annual *Feria Internacional del Turismo* (International Tourism Fair) in Madrid. Along the aisles of this fair, there are various companies that have identified the tourism and health link as a development segment. These include companies that offer care technologies, accessibility for the disabled or for elderly people with disabilities, as well as tour operators that develop a wellness offer. Large health groups have also invested in this sector, such as the Hospiten Group, which manages hospitals and health centers and whose development has followed the growth of Spanish-speaking tourist regions: the Balearic Islands, the Canary Islands and the Riviera Maya in Mexico.

Ultimately, thinking about health within tourism development, from the point of view of the different categories of actors, means integrating health into the tourism offer, either through the services and activities proposed (care and well-being) or through the construction of an argument and a certification of good practices along the lines of what has been done in the environment. Each actor has responsibilities (Table 5.1) in a cross-sectoral effort to certify whole destinations, rather than simply facilities, and thus benefit the local population through indirect spin-offs (health should be an indicator to be taken into account in certification).

	Tourism professionals	Health professionals	Local authorities
Sending location	Providing informed information Encouraging responsible behavior (prevention)	Providing informed information Health preparation for the trip (prevention)	Regulating the relevant sectors (such as travel and transportation) by reinforcing the standards related to health and health risk management
Destination	Ensuring different aspects of health (such as food security, water, sanitation and transportation) Including health in the social and environmental responsibility of companies	Integrating tourism into health planning Including the specificities of tourism in health policies (such as occupational health), prevention and in epidemiological surveillance	Considering territorial development through tourism by including health impacts Promoting cross-sectoral approaches to health

Table 5.1. *Health responsibility of travel actors, inspired by (Rodriguez-Garcia 2001)*

5.4. Transforming tourism: Goal 3 of the Berlin Declaration

Putting an end to the neglect of "health" in tourism implies an evolution, and there are visible signs that this is happening in initiatives such as Transforming Tourism. In 1999, tourism was included in a list of issues by the United Nations Commission on Sustainable Development, which led to the formulation of objectives in a "2030 Agenda". Following this, a group of non-governmental organizations joined together in the Transforming Tourism initiative in order to defend issues, concerns and objectives in the international debate with a view to enriching the 17 goals of the 2030 Agenda, which were considered too unambitious. This process led to the "Berlin Declaration"[3] in 2017 and the drafting of a compendium on each of the 17

3 http://www.transforming-tourism.org/fileadmin/baukaesten/sdg/downloads/Berlin_Declaration.pdf.

aforementioned goals. For the subject at hand, it is the third goal, "Good Health and Well-Being", that needs to be closely examined. Its compendium was written by L. Jaeger (2017)[4] and recalls in the preamble that Goal 3 of the 2030 Agenda calls for a healthy life for all at all ages and that a key demand in this respect includes the prospect of health coverage for all that guarantees access to essential care, as well as to medical consultations and vaccinations at affordable prices. These goals are linked to other ambitions of the 2030 Agenda such as food security, access to water and sanitation, reducing inequality and fighting discrimination, and there are many ways in which tourism can impact these parameters, as we have demonstrated throughout this book. The signatories of the Berlin Declaration identify issues similar to those outlined in the previous chapters, but, more importantly, they propose ways forward.

These are as follows[5]:

– in order for tourism to promote good health and well-being for all, a comprehensive, cross-sectoral and people-centered approach is needed, which takes local people's as well as tourists' health and safety into account and puts a strong focus on equity in order to ensure that local people are not structurally disadvantaged;

– taxes from tourist spending should be used to improve public healthcare systems, allowing for equity and access, particularly for vulnerable groups, in order to avoid further privatization and inflation of medical costs. It is the duty of governments to discourage a dual system of strong disparities where better quality services are reserved for foreign clients with a higher purchasing power while their citizens often lack access to basic healthcare. Governments in the Global South could set quota regulations, which require a set number of treatments of locals for every foreigner treated there;

– the fact that more and more areas of the world get accessed by tourists can support the development of cures and vaccinations for health risks in the Global South that were earlier of little economic interest for pharmaceutical companies. However, these cures have to be made available and accessible not only to affluent tourists but to everyone at risk;

– governments need to develop and enforce laws regarding bioethical questions with regard to tourism, such as organ trafficking, transplant and fertility tourism to effectively protect vulnerable groups within and beyond their borders in line with relevant international guidelines, such as the UN Convention against Transnational Organized Crime (UNTOC);

4 http://www.transforming-tourism.org/goal-3-good-health-and-well-being.html.
5 Excerpts taken from source cited in previous note.

– there is a growing demand for alternative medicine and wellness treatments. This brings great chances for small-scale authentic tourism products that involve local and indigenous communities and their traditional concepts of medicine, health and well-being (this offer must be considered as a complement to allopathic medicine);

– until today, only a very small part of the world's population has been able to take vacations and to travel internationally. Tourists should bear in mind that, for example, in Europe, the entitlement for paid leave was a long and hard struggle by the Trade Unions for workers' rights to health and recreation. Tourists should critically reflect upon their personal consumer behavior and make sure that it does not infringe on the local population's rights to a healthy and dignified life (tourism professionals have a role to play in spreading this message).

The conclusion reached by the signatories of the Transforming Tourism initiative is optimistic: "Tourism has great potential to foster healthy lives and well-being for tourists and local communities if the risks involved are reduced by effective preventative measures."

Conclusion

Health to Change the Development Paradigm?

The relationship between tourism and health is age old. We might even consider that tourism is largely born from a quest for well-being and health. However, with its development and growing internationalization, this sector can now no longer ignore the fact that it is both dependent on a certain number of health parameters (circulation of diseases, risks, socio-demographic changes) and generates direct and indirect impacts on health (of tourists and populations in the destinations), health systems, occupational health and, more generally, the physical and social environment. However, the relationship between tourism and health is too often reduced to medical tourism, which is only the tip of a huge iceberg whose submerged part constitutes the "neglected of tourism and health".

In western societies, tourism is considered as a factor for improving the quality of life, a healthy activity (that benefits us). In an article published in 1995, Perry and Dietrich contrasted the concepts of quality of life, health and the promotional principles of tourism marketing: the "three or four S's" (sea, sun, sand and sex[1]), by questioning "the health of these activities", which led them to call for a new paradigm for the marketing and promotion of tourism.

The back and forth between health and tourism in this book, which is as exhaustive as possible, and which attempts to not neglect any angle of approach or any theme, leads to a rather similar conclusion. Without claiming to fundamentally renew the paradigms of tourism development, it is now imperative to add a line to them that brings health into the considerations. This is a necessity for tourist destinations, but it is also true for sending countries, which are just as affected (Johnston *et al.*, 2010). Also, the understanding of health that prevails in this

1 According to the authors, sex may or may not be added to the triptych of sea, sand and sun.

perspective is holistic: it encompasses both medical tourism and the health and safety of tourists and local populations, the circulation of diseases, knowledge and health practices and, more broadly, all of the conditions that contribute to the quality of life and well-being. The spectrum is very broad and requires the coordination between tourism and health to be considered as a system. This can be summarized on four levels.

From a medical point of view, efforts to understand and deepen knowledge must focus on the evaluation of the harmful impacts of tourism, on the one hand, and the health benefits, on the other hand. This includes monitoring the health status of local populations and tourists, and more qualitative studies, for example on the potential positive aspects of interculturation, as discussed in section 4.3. Changes in dietary practices, the evolution of hygiene standards and the syncretism of healthcare practices are all evolutions that are accompanying the development of tourism, but are understudied in terms of their consequences for health.

At the social level, tourism can have devastating effects on health, or may conversely constitute a powerful lever for progress in working conditions in the organization of social and healthcare systems. Here, public and private actors in the interconnected sectors of tourism, health and territorial development need to be made aware. The question of the weight of tourist demand remains to be evaluated in this respect. For example, we may question whether a certification that guarantees good health practices would carry significant weight (on the social or environmental responsibility accreditation model).

At the environmental level, surprisingly, health is struggling to establish itself as a component of sustainable development, which it undeniably is. In the field of tourism, research avenues are to be explored in the field of therapeutic landscapes. These environments, which are favorable to health (especially psychological health), are at the intersection of hedonistic and eudemonic narratives, both of which are widely discussed in research on tourism and which refer to wellness, which the World Health Organization defines as "a state of complete physical, moral and social well-being".

Finally, at the economic level, the interactions between tourism and health can be read in terms of risks (the losses linked to the Covid-19 crisis provide a glaring short-term illustration), and also (and perhaps above all) in terms of opportunities. Health and wellness tourism is no longer a simple niche market but an emerging one, and tourism operators have at hand a potential to diversify their activities (and sources of income) or to reorient customer segments. Health, in its positive acceptance, has image and display effects that are largely underestimated in marketing terms. This is all supported by the demographic evolution of the western and Asian worlds, the main suppliers of tourists, both of which are seeing an increase in the proportion of seniors in their populations. The result is a growing connection between the tourism and well-being economy and the silver economy, which is likely to change the nature of the tourism offer to meet the needs of this clientele; and if the necessary services are thought out and planned with a view to also serving the local populations, economies of scale can be envisaged for a development that benefits everyone.

A new development paradigm could then emerge, which would make health indicators (of travelers and local populations) an indicator of progress. A recent study published by the Pacific Asia Travel Association suggests that the global Covid-19 pandemic may well accelerate this process and permanently move health out of the category of tourism development "unthought-of", as its authors are observing "emerging trends in travel and tourism health and hygiene regarding traveler booking behavior and resident sentiment. This means that destination managers and marketers need to rethink, rebuild and reposition their destination health and hygiene focus accordingly."

References

Airault, R. (2000). *Fous de l'Inde : délires d'occidentaux et sentiments océaniques*. Payot, Paris.

Airault, R. (2011). Voyages et risques de décompensations psychiatriques. *ADSP*, 76, 43–45.

Amselle, J.L. (2014). Le tourisme chamanique en Amazonie. *Études*, (2), 33–42.

Andrieu, B. (2007). Du teint hâlé honni au bronzage de rigueur. *Cerveau et psycho*, 22, 54–65.

Andrieu, B. (2011). L'héliothérapie ou le soleil bienfaiteur : soleil, mon meilleur ennemi. *Biofutur*, 323, 23–57.

Ateljevic, I. and Doorne, S. (2004). Theoretical encounters: A review of backpacker literature. In *The Global Nomad: Backpacker Travel in Theory and Practice*, Richards, G. and Wilson, J. (eds). Channel View Publications, Bristol.

Banos, S.R. and de Bernardis, A. (2003). Vaccination priorities. *International Journal of Antimicrobian Agents*, 21, 175–180.

Bar-El, Y., Durst, R., Katz, G., Zislin, J., Strauss, Z., Knobler, H.Y. (2000). The Jerusalem syndrome. *British Journal of Psychiatry*, 176, 86–90.

Bauberot, A. (2008). De la nudité thérapeutique au nudisme, les naturistes français. *Rives nord méditerranéennes*, 30 [Online]. Available at: https://journals.openedition.org/rives/2403.

Bauer, I.L. (2001). Tourism and the environment, the other side of the coin: Environmental impact on tourists' health. *Tourist Studies*, 1(3), 297–314.

Baum, T., Kralj, A., Robinson, R.N.S., Solnet, D.J. (2016). Tourism workforce research: A review, taxonomy and agenda. *Annals of Tourism Research*, 60, 1–22.

Basset, V. (2013). Tourisme et chamanisme : entre folklorisation et revitalisation culturelle ? *Téoros*, 32(1), 133–142.

Belot, A., Grosclaude, P., Bossard, N., Jougla, E., Benhamou, E., Delafosse, P., Guizard, A.-V., Molinié, F., Danzon, A., Bara, S. et al. (2008). Cancer incidence and mortality in France over the period 1980–2005. *Revue épidémiologie et santé publique*, 56(3), 159–175.

Bertaud, C. (2012). La thérapeutique des bains de mer. *La côte de beautée*, 117 [Online]. Available at: http://www.lacotedebeaute.info/article/la-therapeutique-des-bains-de-mer, 13068.php.

Bertrand, G. (2010). Grand Tour (tourisme, touriste). In *Dictionnaire des concepts nomades en sciences humaines*, Christin, O. (ed.). Métailié, Paris.

Bessy, O. (1991). Le tourisme de la Forme : à la croisée de la Santé et du sport. *Les cahiers espaces*, 25, 48–55.

Blaho-Poncé, C. (2013). La chaîne d'accessibilité, pivot de l'accès au Tourisme Handicap. *Téoros*, 32(2), 104–115.

Bochaton, A. (2011). La construction de l'espace transfrontalier lao-thaïlandais. *Espace populations sociétés*, 11(2), 337–351.

Bochaton, A. (2015). Migrations sanitaires et nouveaux enjeux autour la frontière lao-thaïlandaise. *L'Espace Politique* [Online]. Available at: http://journals.openedition.org/espacepolitique/3280.

Bochaton, A. (2019). Intertwined therapeutic mobilities: Knowledge, plants, healers on the move between Laos and the U.S. *Mobilities*, 14(1), 54–70.

Bodin, D., Javerlhiac, S., Héas, S., Robène, L. (2009). De l'émergence des stations balnéaires au tourisme sportif : le mélange des genres à la lueur de l'exemple de la région Bretagne en France. *Téoros*, 28(2), 29–36.

Boiville, G. (2005). Les spas, une nouvelle offre de bien-être. *Espaces*, 288, 5.

Borins, M. (2000). Take holidays – it's good for you. *Canadian Family Physician*, 46, 2372–2374.

Bouchaud, O. (2003). Médecine du voyage. *Médecine/sciences*, 19, 489–490.

Bouhaouala, M. and Biard, E. (2015). Collectivités territoriales : tourisme et sport, un duo gagnant. *Jurisport*, 150, 42–45.

Boukhris, L. and Chapuis, A. (2016). Circulations, espace et pouvoir – penser le tourisme pour penser le politique. *L'Espace Politique*, 28, 2016-1. DOI: https://doi.org/10.4000/espacepolitique.3707.

Bourdin, A. (2008). Gentrification : un "concept" à déconstruire. *Espaces et sociétés*, 1(1/2), 23–37.

Bowler, D.E., Buyung-Ali, L.M., Knight, T.M., Pullin, A.S. (2010). A systematic review of evidence for the added benefits to health of exposure to natural environments. *BMC Public Health*, 10(1), 456.

Brougère, G. (2015). Le corps vecteur de l'apprentissage touristique. In *Le tourisme comme expérience : regards interdisciplinaires sur le vécu touristique*, Decroly, J.M. (ed.). Presses de l'université du Québec, Quebec.

Brundtland, G.H., Khalid, M., Agnelli, S., Al-Athel, S., Chidzero, B. (1987). Our common future. Report, Bruntland Commission.

Bruston, M. (2000). Des bains au tourisme : la tentation de l'eau au début de la troisième république. *Mappemonde*, 58(2), 6–11.

Burris, K. and Kim, K. (2007). Review Tattoo removal. *Clinics in Dermatology*, 25(4), 388–392.

Cabanas, E. and Illouz, E. (2018). *Happycratie – Comment l'industrie du bonheur a pris le contrôle de nos vies*. Premier Parallèle, Paris.

Cabezas, A.L. (2008). Tropical blues: Tourism and social exclusion in the Dominican Republic. *Latin American Perspectives*, 35(3), 21–36.

Caccia, J., Chuat, C., Hennebel, C., Vögele, V., Waefler, N. (2017). Docteur, pourquoi j'ai pris l'avion ? Tourisme chirurgical des résidents suisses : ressources disponibles en cas de complications. Document, Faculté de biologie et de médecine de l'UNIL, Lausanne.

Cañada, E. (2015). *Las que limpian los hoteles, historias ocultas de precaridad laboral.* Icaria Editorial, Vilassar de Dalt.

Cañada, E. (2018). Too precarious to be inclusive? Hotel maid employment in Spain. *Tourism Geographies*, 4(20), 653–674.

Canista, P. (2015). Où en est-on de la reconnaissance de la médecine thermale au niveau européen ? *Presse thermale et climatique*, 152, 113–119.

Caumes, E. (2011). État des lieux. *Les maladies du voyage et d'importation*, 76, 12–16.

Cazes, G. (1989). *Les nouvelles colonies de vacances ? Le tourisme international à la conquête du Tiers Monde*. L'Harmattan, Paris.

Cazes, G. (1992). *Fondements pour une géographie du tourisme et des loisirs*. Bréal, Paris.

Chantre, L. (2013). Entre pandémie et panislamisme. *Archives de sciences sociales des religions*, 163, 163–190.

Charatan, F. (2001). Foreigners flock to Cuba for medical care. *British Medical Journal*, 322, 1198–1198.

Chasles, V. (2011). Se déplacer pour se faire soigner : une mobilité en expansion, généralement appelée "tourisme médical". *Géoconfluences* [Online]. Available at: http://geoconfluences.ens-lyon.fr/doc/typespace/tourisme/TourScient2.htm.

Chasles, V. and Girer, M. (2016). Tourisme médical et santé reproductive : l'exemple de la gestation pour autrui en Inde. *Revue francophone sur la santé et les territoires, tourisme, mobilités et santé*. DOI: https://doi.org/10.4000/rfst.514.

Chatterjee, S. (1999). Compliance of Malaria chemoprophylaxis among travelers to India. *Journal of Travel Medicine*, 6(1), 7–11.

Chen, C.-C. and Petrick, J.F. (2013). Health and wellness benefits of travel experiences: A literature review. *Journal of Travel Research*, 52(6), 709–719.

Chessex, P. (1997). Grand tour. In *Dictionnaire européen des Lumières*, Delon, M. (ed.). PUF, Paris.

Cheung, C. and Law, R. (2001). The impact of air quality on tourism: The case of Hong Kong. *Pacific Tourism Review*, 5, 69–74.

Cheung, I.K. and Wilson, A. (2007). Arthroplasty tourism. *Medical Journal of Australia*, 187(11/12), 666–667.

Clary, D. (1991). La migration de retraite en Floride. *Norois*, 150(1), 127–144.

Cocola-Gant, A. (2018). Tourism gentrification. In *Handbook of Gentrification Studies*, Lees, L. and Phillips, M. (eds). Edward Elgar Publishing, Cheltenham and Northampton.

Coëffé, V., Guibert, C., Taunay, B. (2012). Émergences et diffusions mondiales du surf. *Géographie et cultures*, 82, 61–76.

Coëffé, V., Duhamel, P., Guibert, C., Taunay, B., Violier, P. (2016). *Mens sana in corpore turistico* : le corps “dé-routinisé” au prisme des pratiques touristiques. *L'Information géographique*, 80(2), 32–55.

Coëffé, V., Guibert, C., Taunay, B. (2019). Usages sociaux et spatialités du bronzage en Chine. *EspacesTemps.net* [Online]. Available at: https://www.espacestemps.net/en/articles/usages-sociaux-et-spatialites-du-bronzage-en-chine/.

Cohen, E. (1973). Nomads from affluence: Notes on the phenomenon of drifter-tourism. *International Journal of Comparative Sociology*, 14(1/2), 89–103.

Cohen, E. (1988). Tourism and AIDS in Thailand. *Annals of Tourism Research*, 15(4), 467–486.

Cohen, E. (2013). Tattoo tourism in the contemporary West and in Thailand. In *The Routledge Handbook of Cultural Tourism*, Smith, M. and Richards, G. (eds). Routledge, Abingdon.

Connell, J. (2006). Medical tourism: Sea, sun sand and… surgery. *Tourism Management*, 6(27), 1093–1100.

Connell, J. (2013). Contemporary medical tourism: Conceptualisation, culture and commodification. *Tourism Management*, 34, 1–13.

Cooper, M., Vafadari, K., Hieda, M. (2015). *Current Issues and Emerging Trends in Medical Tourism*. IGI Global, Hershley.

Corbin, A. (2018). *Le territoire du vide : l'occident et le désir de rivage*. Flammarion, Paris.

Cossar, J. (1995). Travellers' health: A medical perspective. In *Health and International Tourist*, Clift, S. and Page, S. (eds). Routledge, Abingdon.

Cribier, F. (1984). La retraite au bord de la mer. La fonction d'accueil des retraités des villes touristiques. *Bulletin de l'Association de Géographes Français*, 61(500), 133–139.

Crooks, V.A., Kingsbury, P., Snyder, J., Johnston, R. (2010). What is known about the patient's experience of medical tourism? A scoping review. *BMC Health Services Research*, 10(1), 266.

Dahlgren, G. and Whitehead, M. (1991). Policies and strategies to promote social equity in health. Working document, Institute for Futures Studies, Stockholm.

De Schryver, A. and Meheus, A. (1989). International travel and sexually transmitted diseases. *World Health Statistics Quarterly*, 42(2), 90–99.

Dehoorne, O., Saffache, P., Tatar, C. (2008). Le tourisme international dans le monde : logiques des flux et confins de la touristicité. *Études caribéennes*. DOI: https://doi.org/10.4000/etudescaribeennes.882.

Demanget, M. (2015). Chamanisme, ethnologie et tourisme : le partage du bonheur en question. In *Ethnologie des gens heureux*, Berthon, S., Chatelain, S., Ottavi, M.-N., Wathelet, O. (eds). MSH, Paris.

Demeyère, C. (2020). Tourisme post COVID-19, conditions de travail et précarité dans le secteur touristique. *Téoros* [Online]. Available at: https://journals.openedition.org/teoros/7457.

Dioko, L.D.A. and Harrill, R. (2019). Killed while traveling – Trends in tourism-related mortality, injuries, and leading causes of tourist deaths from published English news reports, 2000–2017. *Tourism Management*, 70, 103–123.

Duhamel, P. (2018). *Géographie du tourisme et des loisirs : dynamiques, acteurs, territoires*. Armand Colin, Paris.

Dutray, B. and Moulin, S. (2005). L'Inde bouleversante : manifestations psychiques au cours des voyages touristiques. *L'Autre*, 6(1), 59–69.

Eades, J. (2015). The growth of medical tourism: Recent trends and issues. In *Current Issues and Emerging Trends in Medical Tourism*, Cooper, M., Vafadari, K., Hieda, M. (eds). IGI Global, Hershey.

Eaker, E.D., Pinsky, J., Castelli, W.P. (1992). Myocardial infarction and coronary death among women: Psychosocial predictors from a 20-year follow-up of women in the Framingham study. *American Journal of Epidemiology*, 135, 854–864.

Équipe MIT (2011). *Tourismes 3, la révolution durable*. Belin, Paris.

Escobar, E.R., Gamiño, M.N.B., Salazar, R.M., Hernández, I.S.S., Martínez, V.C., Bautista, C.F., López, M.G., Buenabad, N.A., Medina-Mora, M.E., Velázquez, J.A.V. (2018). National trends in alcohol consumption in Mexico: Results of the national survey on drug, alcohol and tobacco consumption 2016–2017. *Salud Mental*, 1(41), 7–16.

Eytan, A. and Loutan, L. (2006). Voyages et problèmes psychiatriques. *Revue médicale suisse*, 65(9), 1251–1255.

Fleuret, S. (2020). Développer un territoire par le tourisme revient-il également à un développement dans le champ de la santé ? *Carnets de géographes*, 14.

Fleuret, S. and Atkinson, S. (2007). Wellbeing, health and geography: A critical review and research agenda. *New Zealand Geographer*, 63(2), 106–118.

Fleuret, S. and Jouault, S. (2019). Pour une approche conjointe du tourisme et de la santé : postulats à partir de l'exemple de Cancún – Riviera Maya (Mexique). *Téoro*, 38, 2.

Fleuret, S. and Marie-dit-Chirot, C. (2020). Vivir y malvivir en el país de las vacaciones: desarrollo turístico y salud mental en Quintana Roo, México. *Alba Sud* [Online]. Available at: https://www.albasud.org/noticia/es/1282/vivir-y-malvivir-en-el-pais-de-las-vacaciones-desarrollo-turistico-y-salud-mental-en-quintana-roo-mexico.

Folliard, T. (2008). Phytothérapie externe en Amérique du Sud et en Amérique centrale – Mexique et Guatemala. *Phytothérapie*, 6(3), 175–183.

Fontaine, D. and Bernard, M. (2011). L'offre de médecine générale et la saisonnalité dans les zones touristiques alpines de Rhône-Alpes. Working document, ORS Rhône Alpes, Lyon [Online]. Available at: http://www.ors-auvergne-rhone-alpes.org/pdf/Offredesoins_saisonniers_plaquette.pdf.

Galliot, S. (2009). Un rite de passage polynésien : le tatouage samoan. *Corps*, 6(1), 77–94.

Gardiner, V. (1996). La pollution des plages à Malte. *Méditerranée*, 84, 53–56.

Gautret, P., Schlagenhauf, P., Gaudart, J., Castelli, F., Brouqui, P., von Sonnenburg, F., Loutan, L., Parola, P., GeoSentinel Surveillance Network (2009). Multicenter EuroTravNet/GeoSentinel study of travel-related infectious diseases in Europe. *Emerging Infectious Diseases*, 15(11), 1783–1790.

Gayral, A.M. (2010). *Adapter l'offre touristique aux handicaps. Étude de marché : la population des personnes en situation de handicap et l'offre touristique française.* Atout France, Paris.

Gélard, M.-L. (2014). Les "Bains de sable" dans le Tafilalt. In *Vivre le sable ! Corps, matière et sociétés*, Boulay, S. and Gélard, M.-L. (eds). Maison des Sciences de L'homme, Paris.

Genton, B. and D'Acremont, V. (2018). Travel Apps : applications et sites web en médecine des voyages. *Revue médicale suisse*, 14(605), 938–940.

Gesler, W.M. (1992). Therapeutic landscapes: Medical issues in light of the new cultural geography. *Social Science & Medicine*, 34(7), 735–746.

Ginolin, O. (2004). L'artisanat traditionnel en Polynésie française : de l'économie touristique à l'élaboration des identités insulaires. *Journal de la société des océanistes*, 119, 172–184.

Gladwell, N.J. and Bedini, L.A. (2004). In search of lost leisure: The impact of caregiving on leisure travel. *Tourism Management*, 6(25), 685–693.

Gössling, S. (2005). Tourism's contribution to global environmental change: Space, energy, disease and water. In *Tourism Recreation and Climate Change: International Perspectives*, Hall, C.M. and Higham, J. (eds). Channel View Publications, Bristol.

Grandvoinnet, P. (2010). Histoire des sanatoriums en France (1915–1945) – Une architecture en quête de rendement thérapeutique. PhD Thesis, Universités de Genève and Versailles-Saint Quentin en Yvelines.

Guérin-Beauvois, M. (2000). Les pratiques du thermalisme dans les villes de l'Italie romaine. *Histoire urbaine*, 1(1), 123–144.

Haley, A.J., Snaith, T., Miller, G. (2005). The social impacts of tourism a case study of Bath, UK. *Annals of Tourism Research*, 32(3), 647–668.

Halioua, B., Prazuck, T., Malkin, J.E. (1997). Maladies sexuellement transmissibles et voyages. *Médecine tropicale*, 57, 501–504.

Hallem, Y. and Barth, I. (2011). Étude ethnographique du rôle d'Internet dans le développement du tourisme médical : cas du tourisme de chirurgie esthétique en Tunisie. Working document, École de Management de Strasbourg, Strasbourg.

Hartmann, L. (2009). Les indicateurs de performance des systèmes de santé. *Réalités cardiologiques*, 254, 11–19.

Hartwell, H., Hemingway, A., Fyall, A., Filimonau, V., Wall, S. (2012). Tourism engaging with the public health agenda: Can we promote "wellville" as a destination of choice? *Public Health*, 12(126), 1072.

Heinze, G., Chapa, G.C., Carmona-Huerta, J. (2016). Los especialistas en psiquiatría en México: año 2016. *Salud Mental de México*, 39(2), 69–76. DOI: 10.17711/SM.0185-3325.2016.003.

Herrick, D. (2007). Medical tourism: Global competition in health care. *National Center for Policy Analysis*, 304, 1–40.

Hobson, J.S.P. and Dietrich, U.C. (1995). Tourism, health and quality of life. *Journal of Travel & Tourism Marketing*, 3(4), 21–38.

Hoerner, J.M. (2008). *Géopolitique du tourisme*. Armand Colin, Paris.

Holda, R. (2015). Tourism for family caregivers. In *Current Issues and Emerging Trends in Medical Tourism*, Cooper, M., Vafadari, K., Hieda, M. (eds). IGI Global, Hershley.

Hoyez, A. (2008). L'Espace-Monde du yoga : une géographie culturelle et sociale de la mondialisation des paysages thérapeutiques. *L'Information géographique*, 72(1), 100–108.

Hunter-Jones, P. (2003). The perceived effects of holiday-taking upon the health and wellbeing of patients treated for cancer. *International Journal of Tourism Research*, 5, 183–196.

Hunter-Jones, P. and Blackburn, A. (2007). Understanding the relationship between holiday taking and self-assessed health: An exploratory study of senior tourism. *International Journal of Consumer Studies*, 31(5), 509–516.

IEDOM (2006). Impact économique de l'épidémie de Chikungunya à la Réunion mesuré fin mars 2006. Working document, IEDOM, Paris.

Jaeger, L. (2017). Goal 3: Good health and wellbeing – Ensure healthy lives and promote well-being for all at all ages, transforming tourism. Working document, Tourism Watch, Berlin [Online]. Available at: http://www.transforming-tourism.org/fileadmin/baukaesten/sdg/downloads/Kapitel/Goal_3.pdf [Accessed 20 April 2021].

Jennings, E.T. (2011). *À la cure les coloniaux : thermalisme, climatisme et colonisation française (1830–1962)*. Presses universitaires de Rennes, Rennes.

Jennings, E.T. (2012). Le club des hauteurs : savoirs, réseaux et stations d'altitude coloniaux. In *Territoires impériaux : une histoire spatiale du fait colonial*, Blais, H., Deprest, F., Singaravélou, P. (eds). Éditions de la Sorbonne, Paris.

Johnston, R., Crooks, V.A., Snyder, J., Kingsbury, P. (2010). What is known about the effects of medical tourism in destination and departure countries? A scoping review. *International Journal for Equity in Health*, 9(1), 24.

Kabak, J. (2004). *Holiday cheer is a challenge for the chronically ill: Tips for coping* [Online]. Available at: www.immunesupport.com.

Kevan, S.M. (1993). Quests for cures: A history of tourism for climate and health. *International Journal of Biometeorology*, 37, 113–124.

Klein, R. (2011). Responsible cruise tourism: Issues of cruise tourism and sustainability. *Journal of Hospitality and Tourism Management*, 18(1), 107–116.

Klein, H.J., Simic, D., Fuchs, N., Schweizer R., Mehra T., Giovanoli P., Plock, J.A. (2017). Complications after cosmetic surgery tourism. *Aesthetic Surgery Journal*, 37(4), 474–482.

Kluger, N., Raison-Peyron, N., Guillot, B. (2008). Tatouages temporaires au henné : des effets indésirables parfois graves. *La Presse Médicale*, 7–8(37), 1138–1142.

Kocasoy, G. (1989). The relationship between coastal tourism, sea pollution and public health: A case study from Turkey. *Environmentalist*, 9(4), 245–251.

Kokabi, A.-R. and NnoMan (2020). Femmes de chambre en grève à l'hôtel Ibis : "La sous-traitance, c'est la maltraitance". *Reporterre* [Online]. Available at: https://reporterre.net/Femmes-de-chambre-en-greve-a-l-hotel-Ibis-La-sous-traitance-c-est-la-maltraitance.

Konu, H., Tuohino, A., Komppula, R. (2010). Lake wellness – A practical example of a new service development (NSD) concept in tourism industries. *Journal of Vacation Marketing*, 16(2), 125–139.

Kruizinga, P. (2016). Health tourism and health promotion at the coast. In *The Routledge Handbook of Health Tourism*, Smith, M.K. and Puczkó, L. (eds). Routledge, Abingdon.

Lanquar, R. (1989). La filière du tourisme de santé. *The Tourist Review*, 4(44), 25–30.

Lazzarotti, O. (1994). La géographie dans la controverse touristique. *Annales de géographie*, 580, 627–650.

Le Bigot, B. (2016). Les migrations hivernales des Européens vers le Maroc : circulations et constructions des espaces de vie. *Autrepart*, 77(1), 51–68.

Le Borgne, C. (2007). Le tourisme médical : une nouvelle façon de se soigner. *Les Tribunes de la santé*, 15(2), 47–53.

Le Bras, M., Mazaudier, E., Bigaignon-Receveur, M.C., De La Brelie, N.S., Becquart, J.P., Longy-Boursier, M. (1992). Épidémiologie et clinique des maladies tropicales d'importation. *La Revue de médecine interne*, 13(3), 205–210.

Le Coz, C.J. (2001). Risques des peintures cutanées ou tatouages labiles au "henné noir". *Revue française d'allergologie et d'immunologie clinique*, 5(41), 504–509.

Le Serre, D. and Chevalier, C. (2013). Quand le vieillissement démographique génère des opportunités : le nouveau marché touristique des seniors français, comment l'appréhender ? *Revue française du marketing*, 241, 39–57.

Leahy, A.L. (2008). Medical tourism: The impact of travel to foreign countries for healthcare. *The Surgeon*, 5(6), 260–261.

Lebreton, L., Slat, B., Ferrari, F., Sainte-Rose, B., Aitken, J., Marthouse, R., Hajbane, S., Cunsolo, S., Schwarz, A., Levivier, A. et al. (2018). Evidence that the Great Pacific Garbage Patch is rapidly accumulating plastic. *Scientific Reports*, 8(1), 1–15.

Lecler, S. (2008). Les vertus de l'eau et le tourisme thérapeutique. *Alternatives Économiques*, 271(7), 52–52.

Leggat, P.A. and Shaw, M.T.M. (2003). Travel health advice for backpackers. *Journal of Travel Medicine*, 10, 340–345.

Leroux, E. (2010). Comportement des seniors et tourisme : l'effet modérateur de la variable santé. *Gérontologie et société*, 135(33), 153–166.

Lohez, M. (2000a). Thermalisme et tourisme : les évolutions récentes en France. *L'Information géographique*, 4(64), 314–321.

Lohez, M. (2000b). Thermalisme, entre tourisme et santé. *Festival international de géographie de Saint Dié des Vosges*, Saint Dié des Vosges.

Lohore, S.G. (2018). Tourisme et santé, mise en production des territoires par le tourisme médical. PhD Thesis, Université de Perpignan, Perpignan.

Lovel, H. and Feuerstein, M. (1992). Editorial introduction: After the carnival: Tourism and community development. *Community Development Journal*, 27(4), 335–352.

Luna García, A. (2019). El migrante en la institución de salud mental: la invisibilización de lo evidente. PhD Thesis, El Colegio de la Frontera Norte, Tijuana.

Lunt, N., Smith, R., Exworthy, M., Green, S.T., Horsfall, D.G., Mannion, R. (2011). Medical tourism: Treatments, markets and health system implications: A scoping review. Working document, Organisation for Economic Co-operation and Development, Paris.

Lüthi, D. (2012). Le compas & le bistouri. Architecture de la médecine et du tourisme curatif : l'exemple vaudois (1760–1940). *Histoire, médecine et santé*, 7, 133–134.

Maller, C., Townsend, M., Leger, L., Henderson-Wilson, C., Pryor, A., Prosser, L., Moore, M. (2008). Healthy parks, healthy people: The health benefits of contact with nature in a park context. *The George Wright Forum*, 2(26), 51–83.

Mansanguan, C., Matsee, W., Petchprapakorn, P., Kuhakasemsin, N., Chinnarat, N., Olanwijitwong, J., Piyaphanee, W. (2016). Health problems and health care seeking behavior among adult backpackers while traveling in Thailand. *Tropical Diseases, Travel Medicine and Vaccines*, 2, 9.

Mantion, S. and Peton, M. (2011). Action internationale en santé et en protection sociale : propositions pour une influence française. Report, Ministère du travail, de l'emploi et de la santé, Paris.

Marguerit, D. and Reynaudi, M. (2015). Quelle place pour la France sur le marché international des soins ? Working document, France Stratégie, Paris.

Martet, G. and Normand, P. (2000). Maladies sexuellement transmissibles et voyages. *Revue française des laboratoires*, 321, 19–24.

Maslow, A.H. (1954). *Motivation and Personality*, 3rd edition. Addison-Wesley, New York.

Matter, M. (2015). Chirurgie à l'étranger : un risque clairement non calculé. *Revue médicale suisse*, 482(11), 1512.

McNamara, M., Murphy, A., Dowler, F., Foley, R. (2020). Blue spaces as resources for health and wellbeing: Comparing indoor and outdoor perspectives. *Revista de Estudios Andaluces*, 39, 8–22. DOI: https://dx.doi.org/10.12795/rea.2020.i39.01.

Menvielle, W. and Menvielle, L. (2013). Tourisme médical : un secteur stratégique pour le développement des États. *Revue internationale et stratégique*, 2, 153–162.

Menvielle, W., Menvielle, L., Tournois, N. (2010). Panorama du tourisme médical : une logique de flux migratoires. *Espaces*, 106, 13.

Michel, F. (2011). Bali (Indonésie) : le patrimoine culturel contre ou avec le développement touristique ? Un paradis en sursis et le risque d'un tourisme de luxe non maîtrisé. *Études caribéennes*, DOI: https://doi.org/10.4000/etudescaribeennes.5385.

Miller-Thayer, J. (2010). Health migration: Crossing borders for affordable health care. *Field Actions Science Reports*, (Special Issue 2) [Online]. Available at: http://journals.openedition.org/factsreports/503.

Mock, C., Lorman, J.D., Goosen J., Joshipura, M., Peden, M. (2004). Lignes directrices pour les soins essentiels en traumatologie. Working document, WHO, Geneva.

Mouchet, J., Carnevale, P., Coosemans, M., Fontenille, D., Ravaonjanahary, C., Richard, A., Robert, V. (1993). Typologie du paludisme en Afrique. *Cahiers de santé*, 93(3), 220–238.

Mulhall, B.P., Hu, M., Thompson, M., Lin, F., Lupton, D., Mills, D., Maund, M., Cass, R., Millar, D. (1993). Planned sexual behaviour of young Australian visitors to Thailand. *Medical Journal of Australia*, 158, 530–535.

Myazhiom, A.C.L., Reichhart, F., Himbert, A. (2013). Vacances et loisirs des personnes en situation de handicap mental. Document, Fédération Française de Sport Adapté and Université de Strasbourg, Paris-Strasbourg.

NaRanong, A. and NaRanong, V. (2011). Les effets du tourisme médical : l'expérience thaïlandaise. *Bulletin de l'Organisation mondiale de la Santé*, 5(89), 317–392.

Neviani-Aston, P. (2000). Third age: A time to travel. Report, Mintel, London.

Neyra, J. (2019). Tourisme alternatif au Mexique [Online]. Available at: http://vinculando.org/en/tourisme-alternatif-au-mexique.html.

Noël-Hureaux, E. (2012). Pratiques touristiques et discours sur la santé : et si on partait en balade ? *Tourisme et apprentissages. Actes du colloque de Villetaneuse du 16 et 17 mai 2011*. Experice, Villateneuse.

OECD (2020). Les actions engagées dans le domaine du tourisme face au coronavirus (COVID-19) [Online]. Available at: http://www.oecd.org/coronavirus/policy-responses/les-actions-engagees-dans-le-domaine-du-tourisme-face-au-coronavirus-covid-19-86db4328/.

ORS Pays de la Loire (2008). Impact de l'afflux estival sur les recours aux soins en Vendée. Working document, ORS, Nantes.

ORS Rhône-Alpes (2009). Étude de l'offre de soins libérale dans les zones touristiques alpines de Rhône-Alpes en lien avec la saisonnalité – Étude qualitative et quantitative auprès des médecins généralistes et des chirurgiens-dentistes. Report, ORS Rhône Alpes, Lyon.

ORS Rhône-Alpes (2010). Étude de l'offre de soins libérale dans les zones touristiques alpines de Rhône-Alpes en lien avec la saisonnalité – Effets de la saisonnalité sur l'activité des médecins généralistes et la densité médicale. Report, ORS Rhône Alpes, Lyon.

Ory, P. (2008). *L'invention du bronzage : essai d'une histoire culturelle*. Flammarion, Paris.

Ota, H. (1988). Voyages et déplacements pathologiques des Japonais vers la France. *Nervure*, 1, 12–16.

Page, S.J. and Meyer, D. (1996). Tourist accidents: An exploratory analysis. *Annals of Tourism Research*, 3(23), 660–690.

Parel-Amini, L., Uçkay, I., Rüegg, E.M., Homsy, A., Pittet-Cuénod, B., Modarressi, A. (2019). Les enjeux du tourisme chirurgical dans le domaine de la chirurgie esthétique. *Annales de chirurgie plastique esthétique*, 4(64), 293–297.

Paris, V. (2012). Les performances comparées des systèmes de santé. *Les Tribunes de la santé*, 2, 43–49.

Pearce, P. (1990). *The Backpackers Phenomenon: Preliminary Answers to Basic Questions*. James Cook University of North Queensland, Townsville.

Pène, P. and Touitou, Y. (2009). 09-03 Sport et Santé. Report, Académie Nationale de Médecine, Paris.

Pepi, N., Grosbost, K., Bonnet, G., Vidal, K. (2005). Le spa vend du bien-être. L'offre de spa mérite d'être clarifiée. De la médicalisation des spas. *Espaces*, 228, 4.

Persianova-Dubrova, A.L., Badalov, N.G., Lvova, N.V., Tupitsyna, I.U., Uianaeva, A.I., Krikorova, S.A., Adilov, V.B., Linok, V.A., Povazhnaia, E.L. (2012). Crenobalneotherapy in Russia. *La Presse thermale et climatique*, 149, 93–102.

Planelles, M. (2018). Le poids des mots et des images dans les textes de promotion touristique. In *Le poids des mots. Hommage à Alicja Kacprzak*, Konowska, A., Woch, A., Napieralski, A., Bobińska, A. (eds). WUŁ, Łódź.

Popkin, B.M. and Gordon-Larsen, P. (2004). The nutrition transition: Worldwide obesity dynamics and their determinants. *International Journal of Obesity*, 28(3), S2–S9.

Pratt, S., Tolkach, D., Kirillova, K. (2019). Tourism & death. *Annals of Tourism Research*, 78, 102758. DOI: https://doi.org/10.1016/j.annals.2019.102758.

Pressman, S., Matthews, K.A., Cohen, S., Martire, L.M., Scheier, M., Baum, A., Schulz, R. (2009). Association of enjoyable leisure activities with psychological and physical well-being. *Psychosomatic Medicine*, 7(71), 725–773.

Proulx, L. (2005). Tourisme, santé et bien-être. *Téoros*, 24(3), 5–11.

Quet, M., Pordié, L., Bochaton, A., Chantavanich, S., Kiatying-Angsulee, N., Lamy, M., Vungsiriphisal, P. (2018). Regulation multiple: Pharmaceutical trajectories and modes of control in the ASEAN. *Science, Technology and Society*, 23(3), 485–503.

Ramírez, K.D.C., Martinez Moreno, O.C., Andrade, J.G.R. (2017). Medical cluster of dental services of the City of Tijuana. A description of its competitive forming and operation. *The International Journal of Business Management and Technology*, 1(1), 38–42.

Ranque, S., Gazin, P., Delmont, J. (2004). Schistosomose et tourisme en pays Dogon, Mali. *Médecine Tropicale*, 64, 31–32.

Rauch, A. (1988). *Vacances et pratiques corporelles*. Presses Universitaires de France, Paris.

Raynal, M. (2019). En Tunisie, un Ehpad à la pointe du tourisme médical. *Slate* [Online]. Avaialble at: http://www.slate.fr/story/181743/tunisie-ehpad-trois-etoiles-maison-retraite-hotel.

Reichhart, F. (2011). *Le tourisme adapté : fondements idéologiques et institutionnels*. L'Harmattan, Paris.

Reichhart, F. and Lomo Myazhiom, A.C. (2013). Quel tourisme pour les personnes handicapées ? Enjeux et pratiques du tourisme adapté. *Téoros. Revue de recherche en tourisme*, 32(32–2), 81–85.

Renouard, Y. (1948). Conséquences et intérêt démographique de la Peste noire de 1348. *Population*, 3, 459–466.

Rey, M. (2007). Infectiologie itinérante. *Antibiotiques*, 9, 226–232.

Rial, J.F. (2020). Comment voyagerons nous après la pandémie ? [Online]. Available at: http://tnova.fr/notes/comment-voyagerons-nous-apres-la-pandemie.

Richards, G. and Wilson, J. (2004). *The Global Nomad: Backpacker Traveler in Theory and Practice*. Channel View Publications, Bristol.

Richez, G. (1992). *Parcs nationaux et tourisme en Europe*. L'Harmattan, Paris.

Richter, L.K. (2003). International tourism and its global public health consequences. *Journal of Travel Research*, 41(4), 340–347.

Riley, P.J. (1988). Road culture of international long-term budget travelers. *Annals of Tourism Research*, 15(2), 313–328.

Rodriguez-Garcia, R. (2001). The health-development link: Travel as a public health issue. *Journal of Community Health*, 2(26), 93–112.

Romagosa, F., Eagles, P.F., Lemieux, C.J. (2015). From the inside out to the outside in: Exploring the role of parks and protected areas as providers of human health and well-being. *Journal of Outdoor Recreation and Tourism*, 10, 70–77.

Rosillon, F., Culot, M., Bosser, C., Vaerewyck, J.-F., Vanderborght, P. (2002). Contribution à l'étude de la qualité bactériologique des eaux de surface à vocation touristique en Wallonie (Belgique). *Cahiers de l'Association Scientifique Européenne pour l'Eau et la Santé*, 1/2(7), 3–14.

Roux, S. (2008). La menace touristique. *Civilisations*, 57, 155–170.

Sanchez, A. (1990). Thermalisme : "l'ordonnance plaisir" ? *Espaces*, 17, 5–12.

Sánchez-Ledesma, E., Vásquez-Vera, H., Sagarra, N., Peralta, A., Porthé, V., Díez, E. (2020). Perceived pathways between tourism gentrification and health: A participatory Photovoice study in the Gòtic neighborhood in Barcelona. *Social Science & Medicine*, 258, 13.

Sathyanarayana, D. and Snehalatha, J. (2011). Contemporary relevance of ayurveda in complete healthcare system. *International Journal of Research in Ayurveda & Pharmacy*, 2(2), 328–333.

Saunders, L.E., Green, J.M., Petticrew, M.P., Steinbach, R., Roberts, H. (2013). What are the health benefits of active travel? A systematic review of trials and cohort studies. *PloS One*, 8(8), e69912. DOI: 10.1371/journal.pone.0069912.

Sceau, R. (1974). Évian-les-Bains, station thermale et touristique. *Géocarrefour*, 1(49), 51–75.

Segal, J. (2008). Is pharmaceutical tourism just around the corner? *General Surgery News*, 44–45.

Sharpley, R. (2014). Host perceptions of tourism: A review of the research. *Tourism Management*, 42, 37–49.

Sicsic, J. (2018). Tourisme et bien-être : les diktats du "happiness" ne sont pas sans risques. *Futuroscopie* [Online]. Available at: https://www.tourmag.com/Tourisme-et-bien-etre-les-diktats-du-happiness-ne-sont-pas-sans-risques_a96089.html.

Smith, M.K. and Diekmann, A. (2017). Tourism and wellbeing. *Annals of Tourism Research*, 66, 1–13.

Smith, M.K. and Puczkó, L. (2008). *Health and Wellness Tourism*. Routledge, Abingdon.

Smith, M.K. and Puczkó, L. (2015). More than a special interest: Defining and determining the demand for health tourism. *Tourism Recreation Research*, 40(2), 205–219.

Smith, G.S., Breakstone, H., Dean, L.T., Thorpe, R.J. (2020). Impacts of gentrification on health in the US: A systematic review of the literature. *Journal of Urban Health*, 845–856.

Sönmez, S., Apostolopoulos, Y., Yu, C.H., Yang, S., Mattila, A.S., Yu L.C. (2006). Binge drinking and casual sex on spring break. *Annals of Tourism Research*, 4(33), 895–917.

Steffen, R., Baños, A., deBernardis, C. (2003). Vaccination priorities. *International Journal of Antimicrobial Agents*, 21(2), 175–180.

Stettler, J. (2018). Le tourisme de santé, une veritable opportunité pour les professionnels [Online]. Available at: https://www.gastrojournal.ch/news/detail/le-tourisme-de-sante-une-veritable-opportunite-pour-les-professionnels/.

Stewart, L. and Leggat, P.A. (1998). Culture shock and travelers. *Journal of Travel Medicine*, 5, 84–88.

Stock, M., Dehoorne, O., Duhamel, P., Gay, J.-C., Knafou, R., Lazzarotti, O., Sacareau, I., Violier, P. (2003). *Le tourisme. Acteurs, lieux et enjeux*. Belin, Paris.

Stonich, S.C. (1998). Political ecology of tourism. *Annals of Tourism Research*, 25(1), 25–54.

Suastika, K., Dwipayana, P., Saraswati, I.M.R., Gotera, W., Budhiarta, A.A.G., Sutanegara, I.N.D., Taniguchi, H. (2011). Prevalence of obesity, metabolic syndrome, impaired fasting glycemia, and diabetes in selected villages of Bali, Indonesia. *Journal of the ASEAN Federation of Endocrine Societies*, 26(2), 159–159.

Sun, J., Zhang, J.-H., Wang, C., Duan, X., Wang, Y. (2019). Escape or stay? Effects of haze pollution on domestic travel: Comparative analysis of different regions in China. *Science of The Total Environment*, 690, 151–157.

Taglioni, F. (2010). Virus-sans-frontières : le chikungunya dans le sud-ouest de l'océan Indien et au-delà. In *Frontières et santé : genèses et maillages des réseaux transfrontaliers*, Duhamel, S. and Moullé, F. (eds). L'Harmattan, Paris.

Tessier, D. (2005). Tourisme et infections transmises sexuellement. *Téoros*, 24(3), 19–24.

Théry, H. and Caron, P. (2019). Cartes. Géographie de l'obésité. *Diploweb* [Online]. Available at: https://www.diploweb.com/Cartes-Geographie-de-l-obesite.html.

Thompson, C.W. (2011). Linking landscape and health: The recurring theme. *Landscape and Urban Planning*, 99(3/4), 187–195.

TRAM (2006). Medical tourism: A global analysis. Report, Tourism Research and Marketing, Brussels.

Transforming Tourism, Monshausen, A., Tremel, C., Plüss, C., Koschwitz, G., Lukow, M. (2016). The 2030 agenda for sustainable development. Working document, Bread for the World/Working Group Tourism & Development (akte)/TourCert/Tourism Watch, Berlin.

Vaguet, A. (2018). La santé globale : biopolitique en territoires. *Revue francophone sur la santé et les territoires* [Online]. Available at: https://doi.org/10.4000/rfst.726.

Vermersch, C., Geoffroy, P.A., Fovet, T., Thomas, P., Amad, A. (2014). Voyage et troubles psychotiques : clinique et recommandations pratiques. *La Presse Médicale*, 43(12), 1317–1324.

Vigneron, E. (1999). *Le territoire et la santé : la transition sanitaire en Polynésie française.* CNRS, Paris.

Vincent, J. (2007). *L'Intrusion balnéaire : les populations littorales bretonnes et vendéennes face au tourisme (1800–1945).* Presses universitaires de Rennes, Rennes.

Vogt, J.W. (1976). Wandering: Youth and travel behaviour. *Annals of Tourism Research*, 4(1), 25–41.

Watin-Augouard, J. (2002). Saga Évian. *Revue des marques*, 33.

Welk, P. (2004). The beaten track: Anti-tourism as an element of backpacker identity construction. In *The Global Nomad: Backpacker Travel in Theory and Practice*, Richards, G. and Wilson, J. (eds). Channel View Publications, Bristol.

Whittaker, A. and Leng, C.H. (2016). "Flexible bio-citizenship" and international medical travel: Transnational mobilities for care in Asia. *International Sociology*, 31(3), 286–304.

WHO (1999). Health Impact assessment: Main concepts and suggested approach – Gothenburg consensus paper. Working document, European Center for Health Policy, Brussels.

WHO (2020). Estimation de la mortalité due à la COVID-19. Working document, OMS, Paris.

Yousfi-Bachir, R. and Schaaper, J. (2017). Les déterminants du risque perçu par le touriste français lors du choix d'une destination touristique : un modèle conceptuel. *Question(s) de management*, 16(1), 49–59.

Zhang, A., Zhong, L., Xu, Y., Wang, H., Dang, L. (2015). Tourists' perception of haze pollution and the potential impacts on travel: Reshaping the features of tourism seasonality in Beijing, China. *Sustainability*, 7, 2397–2414.

Index

S, T

U, V, W

Other titles from

iSTE

in

Science, Society and New Technologies

2022

AIT HADDOU Hassan, TOUBANOS Dimitri, VILLIEN Philippe
Ecological Transition in Education and Research

CARDON Alain
Information Organization of The Universe and Living Things: Generation of Space, Quantum and Molecular Elements, Coactive Generation of Living Organisms and Multiagent Model (Digital Science Set – Volume 3)

ELAMÉ Elosh
Sustainable Intercultural Urbanism at the Service of the African City of Tomorrow (Territory Development Set – Volume 1)

KAMPELIS Nikos, KOLOKOTSA Denia
Smart Zero-energy Buildings and Communities for Smart Grids (Engineering, Energy and Architecture Set – Volume 9)

2021

BARDIOT Clarisse
Performing Arts and Digital Humanities: From Traces to Data (Traces Set – Volume 5)

BENSRHAIR Abdelaziz, BAPIN Thierry
From AI to Autonomous and Connected Vehicles: Advanced Driver-Assistance Systems (ADAS)
(Digital Science Set – Volume 2)

DOUAY Nicolas, MINJA Michael
Urban Planning for Transitions

GALINON-MÉLÉNEC Béatrice
The Trace Odyssey 1: A Journey Beyond Appearances
(Traces Set – Volume 4)

HENRY Antoine
Platform and Collective Intelligence: Digital Ecosystem of Organizations

LE LAY Stéphane, SAVIGNAC Emmanuelle, LÉNEL Pierre, FRANCES Jean
The Gamification of Society
(Research, Innovative Theories and Methods in SSH Set – Volume 2)

RADI Bouchaïb, EL HAMI Abdelkhalak
Optimizations and Programming: Linear, Non-linear, Dynamic, Stochastic and Applications with Matlab
(Digital Science Set – Volume 1)

2020

BARNOUIN Jacques
The World's Construction Mechanism: Trajectories, Imbalances and the Future of Societies
(Interdisciplinarity between Biological Sciences and Social Sciences Set – Volume 4)

ÇAĞLAR Nur, CURULLI Irene G., SIPAHIOĞLU Işıl Ruhi, MAVROMATIDIS Lazaros
Thresholds in Architectural Education (Engineering, Energy and Architecture Set – Volume 7)

DUBOIS Michel J.F.
Humans in the Making: In the Beginning was Technique
(Social Interdisciplinarity Set – Volume 4)

ETCHEVERRIA Olivier
The Restaurant, A Geographical Approach: From Invention to Gourmet Tourist Destinations
(Tourism and Mobility Systems Set – Volume 3)

GREFE GWENAËLLE, PEYRAT-GUILLARD DOMINIQUE
Shapes of Tourism Employment: HRM in the Worlds of Hotels and Air Transport (Tourism and Mobility Systems Set – Volume 4)

JEANNERET Yves
The Trace Factory
(Traces Set – Volume 3)

KATSAFADOS Petros, MAVROMATIDIS Elias, SPYROU Christos
Numerical Weather Prediction and Data Assimilation (Engineering, Energy and Architecture Set – Volume 6)

KOLOKOTSA Denia, KAMPELIS Nikos
Smart Buildings, Smart Communities and Demand Response (Engineering, Energy and Architecture Set – Volume 8)

MARTI Caroline
Cultural Mediations of Brands: Unadvertization and Quest for Authority (Communication Approaches to Commercial Mediation Set – Volume 1)

MAVROMATIDIS Lazaros E.
Climatic Heterotopias as Spaces of Inclusion: Sew Up the Urban Fabric (Research in Architectural Education Set – Volume 1)

MOURATIDOU Eleni
Re-presentation Policies of the Fashion Industry: Discourse, Apparatus and Power (Communication Approaches to Commercial Mediation Set – Volume 2)

SCHMITT Daniel, THÉBAULT Marine, BURCZYKOWSKI Ludovic
Image Beyond the Screen: Projection Mapping

VIOLIER Philippe, with the collaboration of TAUNAY Benjamin
The Tourist Places of the World
(Tourism and Mobility Systems Set – Volume 2)

2019

BRIANÇON Muriel
The Meaning of Otherness in Education: Stakes, Forms, Process, Thoughts and Transfers
(Education Set – Volume 3)

DESCHAMPS Jacqueline
Mediation: A Concept for Information and Communication Sciences
(Concepts to Conceive 21st Century Society Set – Volume 1)

DOUSSET Laurent, PARK Sejin, GUILLE-ESCURET Georges
Kinship, Ecology and History: Renewal of Conjunctures
(Interdisciplinarity between Biological Sciences and Social Sciences Set – Volume 3)

DUPONT Olivier
Power
(Concepts to Conceive 21st Century Society Set – Volume 2)

FERRARATO Coline
Prospective Philosophy of Software: A Simondonian Study

GUAAYBESS Tourya
The Media in Arab Countries: From Development Theories to Cooperation Policies

HAGÈGE Hélène
Education for Responsibility
(Education Set – Volume 4)

LARDELLIER Pascal
The Ritual Institution of Society
(Traces Set – Volume 2)

LARROCHE Valérie
The Dispositif
(Concepts to Conceive 21st Century Society Set – Volume 3)

LATERRASSE Jean
Transport and Town Planning: The City in Search of Sustainable Development

LENOIR Virgil Cristian
Ethically Structured Processes
(Innovation and Responsibility Set – Volume 4)

LOPEZ Fanny, PELLEGRINO Margot, COUTARD Olivier
Local Energy Autonomy: Spaces, Scales, Politics
(Urban Engineering Set – Volume 1)

METZGER Jean-Paul
Discourse: A Concept for Information and Communication Sciences
(Concepts to Conceive 21st Century Society Set – Volume 4)

MICHA Irini, VAIOU Dina
Alternative Takes to the City
(Engineering, Energy and Architecture Set – Volume 5)

PÉLISSIER Chrysta
Learner Support in Online Learning Environments

PIETTE Albert
Theoretical Anthropology or How to Observe a Human Being
(Research, Innovative Theories and Methods in SSH Set – Volume 1)

PIRIOU Jérôme
The Tourist Region: A Co-Construction of Tourism Stakeholders
(Tourism and Mobility Systems Set – Volume 1)

PUMAIN Denise
Geographical Modeling: Cities and Territories
(Modeling Methodologies in Social Sciences Set – Volume 2)

WALDECK Roger
Methods and Interdisciplinarity
(Modeling Methodologies in Social Sciences Set – Volume 1)

2018

BARTHES Angela, CHAMPOLLION Pierre, ALPE Yves
Evolutions of the Complex Relationship Between Education and Territories
(Education Set – Volume 1)

BÉRANGER Jérôme
The Algorithmic Code of Ethics: Ethics at the Bedside of the Digital Revolution
(Technological Prospects and Social Applications Set – Volume 2)

DUGUÉ Bernard
Time, Emergences and Communications
(Engineering, Energy and Architecture Set – Volume 4)

GEORGANTOPOULOU Christina G., GEORGANTOPOULOS George A.
Fluid Mechanics in Channel, Pipe and Aerodynamic Design Geometries 1
(Engineering, Energy and Architecture Set – Volume 2)

GEORGANTOPOULOU Christina G., GEORGANTOPOULOS George A.
Fluid Mechanics in Channel, Pipe and Aerodynamic Design Geometries 2
(Engineering, Energy and Architecture Set – Volume 3)

GUILLE-ESCURET Georges
Social Structures and Natural Systems: Is a Scientific Assemblage Workable?
(Social Interdisciplinarity Set – Volume 2)

LARINI Michel, BARTHES Angela
Quantitative and Statistical Data in Education: From Data Collection to Data Processing
(Education Set – Volume 2)

LELEU-MERVIEL Sylvie
Informational Tracking
(Traces Set – Volume 1)

SALGUES Bruno
Society 5.0: Industry of the Future, Technologies, Methods and Tools
(Technological Prospects and Social Applications Set – Volume 1)

TRESTINI Marc
Modeling of Next Generation Digital Learning Environments: Complex Systems Theory

2017

ANICHINI Giulia, CARRARO Flavia, GESLIN Philippe, GUILLE-ESCURET Georges
Technicity vs Scientificity – Complementarities and Rivalries (Interdisciplinarity between Biological Sciences and Social Sciences Set – Volume 2)

DUGUÉ Bernard
Information and the World Stage – From Philosophy to Science, the World of Forms and Communications (Engineering, Energy and Architecture Set – Volume 1)

GESLIN Philippe
Inside Anthropotechnology – User and Culture Centered Experience (Social Interdisciplinarity Set – Volume 1)

GORIA Stéphane
Methods and Tools for Creative Competitive Intelligence

KEMBELLEC Gérald, BROUDOUS EVELYNE
Reading and Writing Knowledge in Scientific Communities: Digital Humanities and Knowledge Construction

MAESSCHALCK Marc
Reflexive Governance for Research and Innovative Knowledge (Responsible Research and Innovation Set - Volume 6)

PARK Sejin, GUILLE-ESCURET Georges
Sociobiology vs Socioecology: Consequences of an Unraveling Debate (Interdisciplinarity between Biological Sciences and Social Sciences Set – Volume 1)

PELLÉ Sophie
Business, Innovation and Responsibility (Responsible Research and Innovation Set – Volume 7)

2016

BRONNER Gérald
Belief and Misbelief Asymmetry on the Internet

EL FALLAH SEGHROUCHNI Amal, ISHIKAWA Fuyuki, HÉRAULT Laurent, TOKUDA Hideyuki
Enablers for Smart Cities

GIANNI Robert
Responsibility and Freedom
(Responsible Research and Innovation Set – Volume 2)

GRUNWALD Armin
The Hermeneutic Side of Responsible Research and Innovation
(Responsible Research and Innovation Set – Volume 5)

LAGRAÑA Fernando
E-mail and Behavioral Changes: Uses and Misuses of Electronic Communications

LENOIR Virgil Cristian
Ethical Efficiency: Responsibility and Contingency
(Responsible Research and Innovation Set – Volume 1)

MAESSCHALCK Marc
Reflexive Governance for Research and Innovative Knowledge
(Responsible Research and Innovation Set – Volume 6)

PELLÉ Sophie, REBER Bernard
From Ethical Review to Responsible Research and Innovation
(Responsible Research and Innovation Set – Volume 3)

REBER Bernard
Precautionary Principle, Pluralism and Deliberation: Sciences and Ethics
(Responsible Research and Innovation Set – Volume 4)

VENTRE Daniel
Information Warfare – 2nd edition

Printed and bound by CPI Group (UK) Ltd, Croydon, CR0 4YY
13/09/2026
14961329-0001